The Bone and Mineral Manual

A Practical Guide

The Bone and Mineral Manual

A Practical Guide

Editors

Michael Kleerekoper
Wayne State University
Detroit, Michigan

Ethel S. Siris
Columbia University
College of Physicians and Surgeons
New York, New York

Michael McClung
Oregon Osteoporosis Center
Portland, Oregon

Academic Press
San Diego   London   Boston   New York   Sydney   Tokyo   Toronto

Cover photo: Scanning electron micrograph of an osteoporotic vertebral trabecular bone.

This book is printed on acid-free paper. ∞

Academic Press
a division of Harcourt Brace & Company
525 B Street, Suite 1900, San Diego, California 92101-4495, USA
http://www.apnet.com

Academic Press
24-28 Oval Road, London NW1 7DX, UK
http://www.hbuk.co.uk/ap/

Library of Congress Catalog Card Number: 98-83212

International Standard Book Number: 0-12-412650-2

PRINTED IN THE UNITED STATES OF AMERICA
99 00 01 02 03 04 EB 9 8 7 6 5 4 3 2 1

To the memory of
John G. Haddad, Jr., 1937–1997
Mentor, colleague, friend

Contents

*Deceased

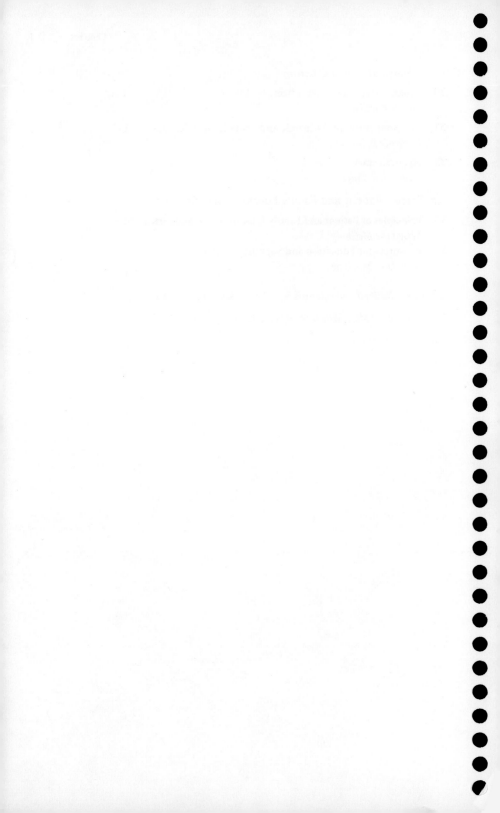

Contributors

John P. Bilezikian, MD
Division of Endocrinology
Department of Medicine
Columbia University
College of Physicians and Surgeons
New York, New York 10032

Albert C. Clairmont, MD
Department of Physical Medicine and Rehabilitation
Ohio State University Medical Center
Columbus, Ohio 43210

Jack W. Coburn, MD
Nephrology Section
University of California, Los Angeles
Los Angeles, California 90073

Murray J. Favus, MD
Department of Medicine
University of Chicago
Pritzker School of Medicine
Chicago, Illinois 60637

Ignac Fogelman, MD
Department of Nuclear Medicine
Guy's Hospital
London, United Kingdom SE1 9RT

Robert F. Gagel, MD
Section of Endocrine Neoplasia and Hormonal Disorders
The University of Texas Medical Center
MD Anderson Cancer Center
Houston, Texas 77030

Harry K. Genant, MD
Osteoporosis and Arthritis Research Group
University of California, San Francisco
San Francisco, California 94143

Susan L. Greenspan, MD
Osteoporosis Prevention and Treatment Center
Beth Israel Deaconess Medical Center
Boston, Massachusetts 02215

John G. Haddad, Jr.*

Hunter Heath III, MD
US Medical Division
Eli Lilly and Company
Indianapolis, Indiana 46285

Frederick S. Kaplan, MD
Department of Orthopaedic Surgery
The University of Pennsylvania School of Medicine
Philadelphia, Pennsylvania 19104

Michael Kleerekoper, MD
Division of Endocrinology
Wayne State University
School of Medicine
Detroit, Michigan 48201

Anne Klibanski, MD
Neuroendocrine Unit
Harvard Medical School
Boston, Massachusetts 02114

Winston Koo, MD
Departments of Pediatrics and Obstetrics/Gynecology
Wayne State University
School of Medicine
Detroit, Michigan 48201

Marjorie Luckey, MD
Saint Barnabas Osteoporosis and Metabolic Bone Disease Center
Livingston, New Jersey
Mount Sinai Medical Center
New York, New York 10014

Barbara P. Lukert, MD
Division of Endocrinology, Metabolism and Genetics
University of Kansas Medical Center
Kansas City, Kansas 66103

Lawrence E. Mallette, MD
Baylor College of Medicine
Houston, Texas 77030

*Deceased

Robert Marcus, MD
Veterans Affairs Medical Center
Palo Alto, California 93405

Velimir Matkovic, MD
Department of Physical Medicine and Rehabilitation
Ohio State University Medical Center
Columbus, Ohio 43210

Betsy Love McClung, RN
Oregon Osteoporosis Center
Portland, Oregon 97213

Michael McClung, MD
Oregon Osteoporosis Center
Portland, Oregon 97213

Karen K. Miller, MD
Department of Medicine
Harvard Medical School
Boston, Massachusetts 02114

Dorothy A. Nelson, MD
Rheumatology Division
Wayne State University
School of Medicine
Detroit, Michigan 48201

Eric Orwoll, MD
Oregon Health Sciences University
Portland VA Medical Center
Portland, Oregon 97201

Jorge A. Prada, MD
Pediatric Bone Center
University of Cincinnati
Cincinnati, Ohio 45267

Robert R. Recker, MD
Center for Osteoporosis Research
Creighton University
Omaha, Nebraska 68131

Elizabeth Shane, MD
Department of Medicine
Columbia University
College of Physicians and Surgeons
New York, New York 10032

Jay R. Shapiro, MD
Uniformed Services University of Health Sciences
Walter Reed Army Medical Center
Washington, District of Columbia 20307

Frederick R. Singer, MD
John Wayne Cancer Institute
Santa Monica, California 90404

Ethel S. Siris, MD
Department of Medicine
Columbia University
College of Physicians and Surgeons
New York, New York 10032

Rebecca L. Slayton, DDS
Department of Pediatric Dentistry
University of Iowa
Iowa City, Iowa 52242

Paul Sponsellor, MD
Department of Orthopedic Surgery
Johns Hopkins University
Baltimore, Maryland 21224

Reginald C. Tsang, MD
Pediatric Bone Center
University of Cincinnati
Cincinnati, Ohio 45267

Nelson B. Watts, MD
Osteoporosis Program
The Emory Clinic
Atlanta, Georgia 30322

Michael P. Whyte, MD
Division of Bone and Mineral Diseases
Washington University School of Medicine
Metabolic Research Unit
St. Louis, Missouri 63131

Preface

Clinical disorders of bone and mineral metabolism have not been extensively taught to medical students or to residents for a number of reasons. Not only was there a limited supply of interested and capable teachers, but the technology for diagnosis and therapeutic options was limited. The rapid growth of awareness of osteoporosis as a major community health problem has changed that dramatically over the past five to ten years. In many arenas, the level of understanding of clinical disorders in this field other than osteoporosis lags far behind. Yet as more clinicians become actively involved in osteoporosis, they are faced on an almost daily basis with clinical scenarios in the field of bone and mineral disorders that are not simply osteoporosis.

Many excellent texts, particularly the *Primer on the Metabolic Bone Diseases and Disorders of Mineral Metabolism* published by the American Society for Bone and Mineral Research, have been published. However, they are generally voluminous and require a substantial effort in order to find out just what to do with the patient lying in the hospital bed or sitting across from you in your office. It is the express purpose of *The Bone and Mineral Manual* to fill that gap by providing a quick and ready reference for immediate handling of both simple and complex clinical disorders of bone and mineral metabolism. We have deliberately truncated background information; that has been left to the larger texts, which must be consulted for in-depth understanding of what might be happening to your patient. Rather, this is a "how-to" manual intended for frequent use while the patient encounter is still in progress.

The book addresses clinical problems likely to be seen at all ages from the preterm infant to the centenarian. As such, it is intended for primary care physicians, but the simple summaries, investigation algorithms, and treatment precis should be of value to the busy specialist for whom this field is not the primary area of specialty focus.

The book has had a long gestation with several updates during preparation to keep current in this fast moving field. We are indebted to the many contributors who agreed with our feeling of the need for such a manual and volunteered their time to provide the initial material and necessary updates. We anticipate the need to return often to these colleagues as we strive to maintain this manual as a living text never outpaced by the knowledge explosion.

Part One

Diagnostic Procedures

1

A Practical Guide
to Bone Densitometry

Dorothy A. Nelson
Michael Kleerekoper

Methods and Measurement Sites

- Dual-energy x-ray absorptiometry (DXA)
  - Lumbar spine, proximal femur, radius/ulna, whole body, phalanges, calcaneus
- Radiographic absorptiometry (RA)
  - Phalanges
- Quantitative computed tomography (QCT)
  - Any region, usually vertebral body
- Single-energy x-ray or photon absorptiometry (SXA, SPA)
  - Calcaneus, radius/ulna
- Broadband ultrasound attenuation (BUA)
  - Sites with thin, uniform soft tissue—calcaneus, tibia

Accuracy and Precision

- Accuracy: how close a measurement is to the true value
- Precision: repeatability of a measurement
- Expressed as percent error using coefficient of variation percent (CV%)
- Varies by method
- Accuracy ranges from 3% to 8%
- Precision ranges from 1% to 5%

Units of Measure

- Bone mineral content (BMC) in grams
- Area (cm^2) or volume (cm^3)
- Bone mineral density (BMD) in g/cm^2 or g/cm^3
- Z-scores and T-scores
  - Standardized scores based on comparison with age-matched (Z) or young adult (T) reference data

The Bone and Mineral Manual
Copyright ©1999 by Academic Press
All rights of reproduction in any form reserved.

Diagnosis of Osteoporosis

• Based on BMD measurement at any skeletal site
• World Health Organization criteria
  – Normal: T-score > –1.0
  – Low bone mass (osteopenia): T-score <–1 but >–2.5
  – Osteoporosis: T-score <–2.5
  – Severe (established) osteoporosis: T-score <–2.5 in the presence of one or more fragility fractures

Who Should Have a Bone Mass Measurement?

• Patients of any age, sex, or ethnicity—if the results will influence a clinical decision

Who Does Not Need a Bone Mass Measurement?

• Healthy premenopausal women
• Healthy young men
• Postmenopausal women already on hormone replacement
• Very elderly and frail patients

How Often Should a Bone Mass Measurement Be Repeated?

• In general, no more often than once every 1 to 2 years
• Less often in women on hormone replacement or other appropriate pharmaceutical therapy
• More often in patients with possible accelerated bone loss (e.g., corticosteroid therapy)

What Rate of Bone Loss Can Be Reliably Detected by DXA?

• The annual bone loss rate is approximately equal to the percentage error in the measurements (1–2%).
• A measured change in bone density should be >2.8 times the error of the measurement, for the clinician to have confidence that this change is real.

2

Indications for Bone Mass Measurement

Dorothy A. Nelson
Michael Kleerekoper

Premenopausal Women

• Any history of medical condition potentially associated with bone loss
  – Secondary amenorrhea
    - anorexia/bulimia
    - excessive exercise
  – Malabsorption (nontropical sprue)
  – Primary hyperparathyroidism
  – Hyperthyroidism
  – Chronic renal failure
• Any history of surgery that might result in bone loss
  – Gastric or intestinal resection
  – Oophorectomy
  – Transplantation
• Any chronic therapy with drugs known to accelerate bone loss
  – Corticosteroids
  – Cyclosporine A
  – Heparin/coumadin
  – Thyroxine
  – GnRH agonists
• Unexplained fragility fractures
  – Stress fractures
  – Vertebral fracture noted incidentally

Early Postmenopause (0–5 years)[1]

• Any of the above indications
• Unwilling or unable to take estrogen
• Undecided about estrogen therapy
• Vertebral deformity on radiograph

The Bone and Mineral Manual
Copyright ©1999 by Academic Press

Late Postmenopause (>65 Years) Not on ERT/HRT[1,2]

• All women

Late Postmenopause (>65 Years) on ERT/HRT

• If any of the premenopausal or early postmenopausal indications have occurred since therapy started

Postmenopause on Therapy for Prevention or Treatment of Osteoporosis

• Estrogen—serial BMD not necessary[3]
• Alendronate—serial BMD at 1 and 3 years of therapy
• Calcitonin—serial BMD at 1 and 3 years of therapy

Men

• Any medical surgical therapeutic history that might be associated with accelerated bone loss
• Fragility fractures

---

1. See also National Osteoporosis Foundation guidelines for bone mass measurement.

2. See also Medicare regulation "Bone Mass Measurement Act" July 1998 for specifics of Medicare reimbursement policies.

3. Many clinicians feel it appropriate to obtain a baseline and followup BMD studies in women who elect to begin ERT/HRT independent of skeletal effects. This is appropriate as is a decision not to obtain BMD measurements.

3

Laboratory Analyses Useful in the Diagnosis of Bone and Calcium Metabolic Disorders

Hunter Heath III

Serum Calcium

- Measure to detect hypercalcemia or hypocalcemia
- Not directly related to bone turnover rates
- Check normal range for lab; should be about 8.9–10.2 mg/dL (2.22–2.55 mmol/L)
- Total calcium is elevated by hyperproteinemia, lowered by hypoproteinemia. Rule of thumb: a change in serum albumin of 1.0 g/dL yields a corresponding change in serum total Ca of 0.8 mg/dL (0.2 mmol/L).
- Tourniquet venous stasis is a very common cause of factitious hypercalcemia; resolve by redrawing blood without a tourniquet.
- Serum-ionized Ca is not altered by changes in serum proteins, but assay is technically difficult and not always available.
- Most common cause of persistent hypercalcemia: primary hyperparathyroidism; second most common: secretion of parathyroid hormone-related protein by malignant tumors
- Most common cause of persistent hypocalcemia: vitamin D deficiency and/or intestinal malabsorption; also common: postsurgical and other forms of hypoparathyroidism

Serum Phosphorus

- Measure to detect effects of poor phosphorus intake, parathyroid hormone excess or deficiency, phosphate retention in renal failure.
- Serum phosphorus levels drop rapidly with lack of oral intake.
- PTH excess decreases serum phosphorus by enhancing renal excretion (decreasing renal tubular reabsorption).
- Serum phosphorus concentrations consistently elevated in hypoparathyroid states (increased renal tubular reabsorption)
- Falsely elevated by hemolysis
- Normal ranges laboratory-specific, and dependent on age

Serum Parathyroid Hormone

- Method of choice: 2-site immunometric assays
  - Immunoradiometric assays (IRMA) use radioactive tracers in test tube.
  - Immunochemiluminometric assays (ICMA) require no radioactivity.
- 2-site assays exquisitely sensitive and specific for intact, biologically active PTH-(1-84)
- These assays can detect not only elevated but subnormal serum PTH levels.
- Older "carboxy-terminal" and "mid-region" assays no longer indicated
- Measure to detect hypercalcemia or hyposecretion of PTH for pathophysiologic diagnosis of hypercalcemia and hypocalcemia.
- Normal ranges similar among assays but laboratory-specific; approximate normal adult range is 10–65 pg/mL (1.06–6.90 pmol/L).
- In primary hyperparathyroidism, serum Ca and PTH levels are positively correlated.
- 10–15% of patients with primary hyperparathyroidism have serum PTH within the normal range, but abnormally elevated for the degree of hypercalcemia.
- In persistent hypercalcemia, serum PTH values below the middle of the normal range strongly suggest something other than primary hyperparathyroidism, such as humoral hypercalcemia of malignancy, familial benign hypocalciuric hypercalcemia, or vitamin D intoxication.
- No clinically meaningful diurnal variation or effect of fasting or feeding
- Serum PTH values are only interpretable with concurrent measurement of serum Ca.

Serum Vitamin D Metabolites

25-Hydroxyvitamin D or Calcediol

- Most useful measurement: 25-hydroxyvitamin D [25(OH)D], because it is the predominant circulating metabolite and best reflection of either nutritional vitamin D deficiency or vitamin D excess
- Normal range approximately 5–80 ng/ml
- There is a pronounced circannual variation in serum 25(OH)D, due to seasonal changes in sun exposure and dermal generation of vitamin D; serum 25(OH)D levels also higher in warm, sunny climates than in northern latitudes.
- Hypercalcemia due to vitamin D intoxication usually associated with markedly elevated serum 25(OH)D values (>200 ng/ml)
- In vitamin D deficiency, serum 25(OH)D levels are generally <5–8 ng/ml, and may be undetectable.

1,25-Dihydroxyvitamin D or Calcitriol

- Calcitriol is the vitamin D metabolite with greatest biological activity, produced from 25(OH)D in kidney, by 25-hydroxyvitamin D 1-alpha hydroxylase.
- Serum calcitriol levels raised by actions of PTH, hypocalcemia, and hypophosphatemia on the hydroxylase enzyme
- Normal range, approximately 20–60 pg/ml (50–150 pmol/L)
- Measurement rarely indicated in clinical practice
- Measure in hypercalcemia only if serum PTH, PTH-related protein, and 25(OH)D are *not* elevated, to detect hypercalcemia due to ingestion of calcitriol, to sarcoidosis and other granulomatoses, or to rare hypersecretion of calcitriol from tumors.
- Serum calcitriol levels are *not* accurate representations of nutritional vitamin D status: levels may be normal in vitamin D deficiency and vitamin D intoxication.

Serum Parathyroid Hormone–Related Protein (PTHrP)

- PTHrP is a normal product of skin, placenta, lactating mammary tissue, and certain neural tissues; mice lacking PTHrP have severe skeletal dysplasias.
- Best assay: 2-site immunometric assays
- Marked variation of normal ranges among assays
- PTHrP levels in normal plasma very low or undetectable
- Measure to diagnose humoral hypercalcemia of malignancy (HHM) due to hyper-secretion of PTHrP by a neoplasm *only* after determining that serum PTH is suppressed.
- Typical biochemical picture in HHM: severe hypercalcemia (often >12.0 mg/dL or >4.0 mmol/L), hypophosphatemia (unless in renal failure), suppressed PTH, normal serum 25(OH)D, low-to-normal serum calcitriol, and elevated PTHrP

Excretion of Calcium and Phosphorus in Urine

- Excretion of Ca in urine varies somewhat with diet but is relatively stable day to day.
- Measure both Ca and creatinine in a 24-hour collection; use creatinine to assess completeness of collection (should be 15–25 mg creatinine/kg body weight).
- Urinary Ca low in: vitamin D deficiency, intestinal malabsorption, very low dietary Ca intakes, familial benign hypocalciuric hypercalcemia
- Urinary Ca elevated in idiopathic hypercalciuria, primary hyperparathyroidism (50% of cases); often strikingly elevated in humoral hypercalcemia of malignancy, vitamin D intoxication (>500 mg/24 hour)
- Measure urinary Ca excretion to evaluate Ca urolithiasis, hypercalcemia, suspected renal Ca leak in osteoporosis, and suspected intestinal malabsorption.
- Urinary phosphorus excretion largely reflects dietary phosphorus intake, and its measurement is seldom of diagnostic value.
- Assessment of urinary phosphorus clearance is of value in assessing chronic hypophosphatemic states to verify that hypophosphatemia is due to renal losses rather than low dietary intake or malabsorption.

Strategy for Pathophysiologic Diagnosis of Hypercalcemia

- Verify that hypercalcemia is persistent and not an artifact due to hyperproteinemia.
- Determine by history any obvious causes (e.g., vitamin D ingestion, immobilization, symptoms of cancer, familial hypercalcemia).
- Measure serum PTH and Ca, 24-hour urine Ca and creatinine.
- If serum PTH is high-normal or elevated, and urinary Ca is normal or elevated, the diagnosis is primary hyperparathyroidism (>90% certainty), and management depends on severity.
- If serum PTH is suppressed to below normal and urinary Ca is high, this is "parathyroid-suppressed hypercalcemia;" measure serum PTHrP and 25(OH)D, which may confirm diagnoses of humoral hypercalcemia of malignancy or vitamin D intoxication.
- If PTHrP is elevated, determine location of tumor and treat appropriately.
- If 25(OH)D is elevated, remove source of exogenous vitamin D; if hypercalcemia is severe, treat with glucocorticoids and low Ca intake.
- If serum PTH is suppressed, urinary Ca is high, and PTHrP and 25(OH)D are normal, measure serum $1,25(OH)_2D$ (calcitriol) to detect rare hypersecretion of calcitriol by tumor or granulomas (e.g., sarcoidosis).
- If serum Ca is high, urine Ca is low (generally, <100 mg/d, often <50 mg/d), and serum PTH, PTHrP, and vitamin D metabolites are normal, consider a diagnosis of familial benign hypocalciuric hypercalcemia, a benign condition due to inactivating (loss-of-function) mutations of the parathyroid cell Ca receptor.

Strategy for Pathophysiologic Diagnosis of Hypocalcemia

- Verify that hypocalcemia is persistent and not due to hypoproteinemia.
- Measure simultaneously serum Ca and PTH.
- If serum Ca and PTH are both low, diagnose hypoparathyroidism and treat appropriately.
- If serum Ca is low and PTH is high, suspect vitamin D deficiency, intestinal malabsorption of Ca, or renal losses of Ca; measure serum 25(OH)D and 24-hour urinary excretion of Ca and creatinine.
- If serum Ca is low, PTH is normal or low, and urinary excretion of Ca is unexpectedly high (e.g., normal in the face of hypocalcemia), suspect the rare syndrome of familial hypercalciuric hypocalcemia due to *activating* mutations of the parathyroid Ca receptor.

How to Interpret the Serum Chemistry Panel in Hypercalcemia and Hypocalcemia

Calcium: severe hypercalcemia (>12–13 mg/dL or >3.0–3.25 mmol/L) should suggest humoral hypercalcemia of malignancy; minimal hypercalcemia often remits without intervention; severe hypocalcemia suggests classical hypoparathyroidism if renal function is normal

Phosphorus: hypophosphatemia is only found in half of primary hyperparathyroid cases, but hyperphosphatemia is much more common in hypoparathyroidism; should be determined in fasting sample to avoid dietary effects

Creatinine: renal failure common in sarcoidosis, vitamin D intoxication, humoral hypercalcemia of malignancy and rare in primary hyperparathyroidism; serum calcitriol levels often low in severe chronic renal insufficiency

Albumin: often low in patients having humoral hypercalcemia of malignancy, chronic renal insufficiency, intestinal malabsorption, malnutrition

Globulins: may be elevated in multiple myeloma

Chloride: generally >103 mEq/L in primary hyperparathyroidism

Cholesterol: generally low in malabsorption causing hypocalcemia

4

Biochemical Markers of Bone Remodeling

Michael Kleerekoper

Biochemical Markers of Bone Remodeling

- Clinical utility
  - Project rate of bone loss
    - high remodeling rate—high rate of loss
    - low remodeling rate—low rate of loss
  - Assess response to therapy
    - substantial reduction in level of markers in patients on anti-resorptive therapy associated with a subsequent increase in BMD
- No well-documented value in predicting bone mass or predicting fracture occurance, except in elderly >age 75

Therefore, markers are adjunctive tests to bone densitometry and not surrogate tests for bone densitometry; they cannot be used as stand-alone tests to diagnose osteoporosis or other metabolic bone disease.

Resorption Markers

- All currently commercially available markers are urine tests and subject to considerable biologic variability.
  - Substantial diurnal rhythm
  - Results must be normalized for urine creatinine excretion.
  - Specimen requirement is either a complete 24-hour collection or first or second void (spot sample) after an overnight fast of at least 6 hours.
- Pyridinium cross-links of type I collagen
  - Pyridinoline (free and bound)
    - PYRILINKS
  - Deoxypyridinoline (free and bound)
    - PYRILINKS-D *(more specific than PYRILINKS)*
- Telopeptides of the cross-links of type I collagen
  - Amino-terminal (NTX)
    - OSTEOMARK
  - Carboxy-terminal (CTX)
    - CROSSLAPS

Formation Markers

- Serum-based assays subject to less biologic variability than resorption markers
- Minimal diurnal variation
- Total serum alkaline phosphatase
  - Limited sensitivity and specificity
  - Inexpensive, widely available
  - Most useful when markedly elevated (>2–3 times upper limit of reference interval), e.g., Paget's disease, osteomalacia, renal osteodystrophy)
- Bone-specific alkaline phosphatase (BSAP)
  - Tandem-OSTASE
    - an immunoradiometric assay with results expressed in mass units
  - Alkphase-B
    - an enzyme immunoassay with results expressed in enzyme activity units
- Osteocalcin
  - Several immunoassays available commercially
    - osteocalcin present in serum as the intact molecule and as a number of smaller fragments
    - different assays detect intact osteocalcin and/or fragments
    - most assays appear to have clinical utility but cannot switch between assays for serial studies in individual patients

Bone Resorption

- Bone resorption is rapid (10 days) and precedes formation which is a much slower process (90+ days).
  - Changes in resorption markers will be apparent more quickly than changes in formation markers.
  - In practice this is of limited importance since changes in formation markers should be detected at a 3-month follow-up visit and earlier follow-up is not generally indicated in patients with metabolic bone disease.

When to Order a Biochemical Marker of Bone Remodeling

- Early menopause, undecided about estrogen therapy, BMD normal
  - High values suggest rapid bone loss and re-thinking of therapeutic decision (reconsider estrogen or consider calcitonin, bisphosphonate, raloxifene) or need for yearly follow-up of BMD.
- Any time postmenopause to help determine whether dose of estrogen is sufficient to retard bone loss
  - Very high baseline value may suggest that higher than average initial dose may be appropriate.
  - High value after three months of therapy
    - problems with compliance
    - need for higher dose or addition of calcitonin or bisphosphonate
- To check effectiveness of nasal spray calcitonin therapy
  - Only 75% of patients in the clinical trials demonstrated an increase in spine BMD.
    - High values for markers when patient is on therapy suggest patient may need higher dose (best first choice) or is a non-responder.
- To check effectiveness of oral bisphosphonate therapy
  - Drugs are only effective if absorbed, and some patients may not be taking therapy exactly as prescribed resulting in no absorption and no therapeutic effect.
  - Very few (<5%) non-responders
    - High values for markers in patients on therapy suggest problems with compliance or that patient has not followed specific instructions for taking the therapy.

What is a High Value for Biochemical Markers?

- Theoretical
  - Any value more than two standard deviations above the mean for the reference population
    - best reference data available for premenopausal white women
- Practical
  - Markers should be evaluated in conjunction with bone density.
    - the lower the bone density, the lower the threshold of concern about biochemical markers as predictors of rates of bone loss
  - Any value in the top quartile of the reference interval
    - remodeling not an all-or-none phenomenon, and the higher the rate of remodeling the greater the rate of loss

What Change in Biochemical Markers Should Be Considered as a Positive Response to Antiresorptive Therapy?

- Theoretical
  - A reduction in the level that is more than can be accounted for by assay and biologic variability
    - 95% confidence that the change is real
- Practical
  - Any reduction 30% or more from the baseline value
    - >80% confidence that the change is real

How Often Should Markers Be Measured?

- In most circumstances baseline and 3-month follow-up are sufficient unless dose of therapy or the disease process has changed.

Advantages of Biochemical Markers

- Specimens can be collected in any physician's office.
- Patients and physicians are used to monitoring disease and response to therapy with laboratory (blood and urine) tests.
- Long-term effectiveness of therapy can be estimated much more quickly (3 vs. 12 months) than by serial measurement of bone density.

Disadvantages of Biochemical Markers

- Limited data demonstrating a relationship between decreasing levels (on therapy) and reduction in fracture occurrence
  - Data for change in BMD and reduction in fracture occurrence more compelling

5

Skeletal Imaging: Radiographs, CT, MRI

Harry K. Genant

Techniques and Applications

- Conventional radiography (all bone disorders)
- (3D)CT (trauma, neoplasms, infection)
- Ultrasound (joints and tendon disease)
- Magnetic resonance imaging (neoplasms, inflammation, infection, joint and tendon disease, bone marrow disorders)
- Arthrography (joint disease)
- Nuclear medicine (inflammation, neoplasm, trauma)

Bone and Mineral Disorders: Radiographic Features

- Osteoporosis (bone loss)
  - Decrease in bone density
  - Cortical thinning
  - Trabecular stress line accentuation
  - Vertebral deformities, wrist and hip fractures
- Osteomalacia (bone mineral loss)
  - Decrease in bone density
  - "Fuzzy" trabeculae
  - "Bowing, buckling" bones
- Osteopenia (decrease in bone density)
  - Regional decrease in bone density
    - disuse, Sudecks's atrophy, transient osteoporosis of the hip, regional migratory osteoporosis
  - Generalized decrease in bone density
    - osteoporosis, osteomalacia, hyperparathyroidism, bone marrow disorders

- Increase in bone density
  - Regional
    - developmental (dysplasia, osteopoikilosis, tuberous sclerosis)
    - neoplastic (myeloma, lymphoma, mastocytosis, metastases)
    - Paget's disease
    - bone infarcts
    - post-trauma
  - Generalized
    - renal osteodystrophy
    - fluorosis, lead poisoning, hypervitaminosis A or D
    - Paget's disease
    - neoplasms (lymphoma, mastocytosis, metastases)
    - dysplasias and hyperostoses

Uses

- Confirming clinical suspected diagnosis
- Providing differential diagnosis
- Screening for disease and disorders
- Monitoring disease regression/progression
- Monitoring therapeutic interventions
- Providing imaging-guided biopsies
- Providing imaging-guided interventions

Scintigraphy

Ignac Fogelman

Advantages

- Provides a functional display of skeletal metabolism
- Highly sensitive for lesion detection
- Rapid evaluation of the total skeleton

Disadvantage

- Appearances are nonspecific.

In Osteoporosis

- Identifies fracture
- Assists in assessing whether a fracture detected by x-ray is new or old
- Bone scan following fracture stays "hot" for 3–9 months in most cases and rarely longer than 18 months.
- Identifies other causes of pain, e.g., facetal joint disease
- Identifies coexistent pathology, e.g., metastases or infection

In Osteomalacia

- Detects pseudofractures
- Suggested by often symmetrical lesions involving multiple ribs (most common site) or pubic ramus, proximal femur/humerus, and scapula.

In Hyperparathyroidism

• Assessment of severity of skeletal involvement by subjective evaluation of metabolic features:
  – Increased tracer uptake in axial skeleton
  – Increased tracer uptake in long bones
  – Increased tracer uptake in periarticular areas
  – Faint or absent kidney images
  – Prominent calvaria and mandible
  – Beading of the costochondral junctions
  – "Tie sternum"
• Identify brown tumors

In Paget's Disease

• Bone scan features
  – Intense uptake of tracer
  – Diffuse involvement of bone
  – Anatomic outlines emphasized, e.g., transverse processes in spine
  – Bone appears expanded, e.g., spine, tibia, humerus
  – Ends of long bone affected
• Earliest evidence of active disease
• Documentation of extent of disease
• May not be able to identify coexistent fracture or sarcomatous change

Bone Biopsy in Malignant and Metabolic Bone Diseases

Robert R. Recker

Pathological Examination of Bone Malignancies

- Bone tumor specimens are obtained from the tumor itself.
- Marrow biopsy specimens are obtained from the posterior iliac crest for diagnosing marrow malignancies.
- Specimens are decalcified and then prepared as soft tissue specimens (paraffin embedding and thin sectioning).
- Standard surgical pathology methods are used for diagnosis.

Transilial Bone Biopsy Is Used to:

- Diagnose metabolic bone disease and bone remodeling abnormalities.
- Evaluate the pathophysiology of metabolic bone diseases (research).
- Assess long-term safety of new bone-active drugs.
- Assess trabecular bone microstructure.

Transilial Bone Biopsy Procedure

- Label with tetracycline prior to biopsy.
- Use tetracycline, 250 mg, q.i.d., 3 days on, 14 days off, 3 days on, then biopsy 5–14 days after the second label. Other labeling schedules may be satisfactory.
- Outpatient setting under local anesthesia
- Obtain the specimen from about 2 cm inferior and posterior to the anterior-superior spine using a trephine at least 7.5 mm in diameter.
- A successful biopsy should produce an intact core including both cortices and the intervening trabecular bone.
- Place the specimen in 70% ethanol as fixative and storage medium.
- Send the specimen in fixative to a reference laboratory. Most hospital pathology laboratories are not able to process bone biopsies, thus arrangements for a reference laboratory must be made prior to biopsy.

Processing by the Reference Laboratory

- The reference laboratory dehydrates, defats, embeds, sections, and reads the specimens without removing the mineral.
- The reference laboratory obtains undecalcified thin sections, 5 mm in thickness, and performs semiautomated quantitative histomorphometry.

Histomorphometric Variables from Trabecular Bone

- Microstructural variables include trabecular number, separation and width, and wall thickness of osteons.
- All other variables incorporate structural measurements and/or trabecular surface measurements.
- The mineral apposition rate (interlabel width/interlabel time interval, MAR) is the key dynamic variable.
- All dynamic variables come from this measurement, i.e., bone formation rates, remodeling periods, and osteoblast work efficiency.
- Osteoid thickness (mm), osteoid surface (%) and MAR are used to calculate the lag time between osteoid deposition and its mineralization. The mineralization lag time (MLT) is the most sensitive variable in detecting osteomalacia.

Prominent Histomorphometric Features of Some Bone Diseases

- Osteoporosis features reduced number, increased separation and normal thickness of trabeculae, and reduced trabecular bone volume.
- Remodeling abnormalities in osteoporosis are subtle and not always identifiable.
- The earliest lesions of mild vitamin D deficiency are increased resorption surface and osteoclast numbers and slight prolongation of the MLT.
- The lesions of severe vitamin D deficiency are thick osteoid seams and absent bone cells.
- The lesions of mild hyperparathyroidism are increased resorption surface and osteoclast numbers, and increased bone remodeling rates (including increased bone formation rates).
- Severe hyperparathyroidism features high remodeling along with fibrous tissue appearing in the marrow space.
- Renal osteodystrophy may feature predominantly hyperparathyroid lesions or osteomalacia lesions, or a mixture of both.
- The "aplastic bone lesion" of renal osteodystrophy is characterized by absent bone cells and absent tetracycline label. There may also be excess osteoid and reduced bone volume.

Indications for Bone Biopsy

Postmenopausal Osteoporosis

- To rule out confounding diagnoses
- To compare with biopsies during treatment
- To determine safety of a test drug (remodeling suppressor)

Vitamin D-Resistant Rickets

- To make the diagnosis
- To judge the success of treatment
- To evaluate the effect of changes in treatment
- To evaluate new treatments

Renal Osteodystrophy

- To diagnose the lesion in symptomatic patients
- To evaluate the success of treatment

Nutritional Rickets and Osteomalacia

- To diagnose the occult form among the elderly

Bone Disease Associated with GI Disease

- To assess bone status in patients with malabsorption or sprue
- To verify the response to treatments

Bone Disease Associated with GI Surgery

- To document the presence of vitamin D deficiency
- To distinguish it from the joint and connective tissue disorders which may accompany GI surgery

Anticonvulsant Osteomalacia

- To diagnose the bone lesion
- To make treatment decisions that avoid fractures

Part Two

Clinical Disorders

8

Hypocalcemia and Hypercalcemia in Neonates

Winston Koo

Neonatal Hypocalcemia

Pathophysiology

Ca	↓ intake or absorption	Prematurity; malabsorption syndrome
iCa	↑ calcium complex	Chelating agent (eg., citrated blood for exchange transfusion, long-chain free fatty acid)
Mg	↓ tissue store or absorption	Maternal hypomagnesemia; IDM specific Mg malabsorption (rare)
P	↑	Endogenous and exogenous (e.g., dietary, enema) phosphate loading
pH	↑	Respiratory or metabolic alkalosis (i.e., shifts Ca from ionized to protein-bound fraction)
PTH	↓ production	Maternal hyperparathyroidism; hypo-parathyroidism; DiGeorge syndrome; hypomagnesemia
PTH	↓ responsiveness	Hypomagnesemia; pseudohypopara-thyroidism
CT	↑	IDM, birth asphyxia, prematurity
$1,25(OH)_2D$	↓ end-organ responsiveness	Prematurity
Activating CaR	↑ responsiveness	Autosomal dominant or sporadic hypocalcemia with hypercalciuria

Ca, calcium; iCa, ionized calcium; Mg, magnesium; P, phosphorus; PTH, parathyroid hormone, CT, calcitonin; IDM, infant of an insulin-dependent diabetic mother; $1,25(OH)_2D$, 1,25-dihydroxyvitamin D; CaR, calcium sensing receptor

Diagnostic Workup

- History
  - Familial
  - Pregnancy (maternal illness, e.g., diabetes mellitus, hyperparathyroidism; intrapartum events; and infant's gestational age)
  - Dietary intake of infant
- Physical
  - Jitteriness
  - Apnea
  - Cyanosis
- Examination
  - Seizures
  - Associated features (infant of diabetic mother, prematurity, birth asphyxia, congenital heart defect)
- Investigations
  - Serum: calcium, magnesium, phosphorus, ionized calcium, glucose, vitamin D metabolites, parathyroid hormone, calcitonin
  - Acid-base balance
  - ECG (Q-Tc > 0.4 sec or Q-oTc > 0.2 sec)
  - Chest x-ray film (thymic shadow, aortic arch position)
  - Chromosomal analysis for 22q11 deletion; molecular genetic studies
  - Others: urine, calcium, magnesium, phosphorus, creatinine, and drug screen; malabsorption workup; maternal/family screening

Management

- Symptomatic hypocalcemia
  - Intravenous: 10–20 mg elemental calcium, e.g. 10% calcium gluconate (9 mg elemental Ca/ml) or 10% calcium chloride (27 mg elemental Ca/ml), infused with dextrose water or normal saline under constant ECG monitoring. Repeat as necessary. Treat hypomagnesemia if present.
  - Continue IV or oral supplement after symptom resolution and until serum Ca is normalized.
- Asymptomatic hypocalcemia
  - Oral: 50–75 mg elemental calcium per kg per day as calcium carbonate (100 mg/ml), glubionate (23 mg/ml), chloride (27 mg/ml) or gluconate (9 mg/ml), in 4 to 6 divided doses until serum Ca normalized for 12–24 hours then decrease supplement by half each 24 hours for 2 days then discontinue supplementation.
  - For infants not receiving mother's milk, a brief period (several weeks) of very low phosphorus milk formula may be useful.
- Genetic counseling as appropriate

Prevention

- Treatment and prevention of underlying disorders
- Early milk feeding or parenteral nutrition

Neonatal Hypercalcemia

Etiology

- Phosphate deficiency
  - Parenteral nutrition
  - Very-low-birth-weight infants fed human milk or (less commonly) standard formula
- Hypervitaminosis D
  - Mother or infant
  - Subcutaneous fat necrosis(?)
- Hyperparathyroidism
  - Congenital parathyroid hyperplasia
  - Maternal hypoparathyroidism
  - Maternal and neonatal renal tubular acidosis
- Prostaglandin-related disorder
  - Bartter syndrome variant
- Mutations in calcium sensing receptor gene
  - Neonatal, severe (primary) hyperparathyroidism
  - Familial, hypocalciuric hypercalcemia
- Uncertain pathophysiological mechanism
  - Extracorporeal membrane oxygenation therapy
  - Idiopathic infantile hypercalcemia (Williams syndrome)
  - Severe infantile hypophosphatasia
  - Blue diaper syndrome
    - congenital hypothyroidism
    - congenital mesoblastic nephroma
- Chronic maternal hypercalcemia (?)
  - Thyrotoxicosis
  - Chronic thiazide diuretic, lithium therapy
  - Vitamin A intoxication

Diagnostic Workup

- History
  - Dietary history (low or no phosphate intake)
  - Medications (excessive vitamin D intake—maternal or infant
  - Perinatal history, e.g., asphyxia
  - Familial or maternal Ca or P diseases
  - Usually asymptomatic or nonspecific, e.g., nausea, vomiting, refusal to feed
- Physical examination
  - Poor growth parameters, lethargy, dehydration, seizures, hypertension, band kerotopathy (rare)
  - Associated features, e.g., elfin facies, congenital heart disease, mental retardation, subcutaneous fat necrosis

• Investigations
  – Serum: calcium, magnesium, phosphorus, ionized calcium, total protein, alkaline phosphatase (total and bone specific), vitamin D metabolites, parathyroid hormone
  – Acid base status
  – Urine: calcium, phosphorus, creatinine, amino acids, cyclic adenosine monophosphate (AMP)
  – Radiographs: chest, hand
  – Determination of hypercalcemic effects: renal function, abdominal ultrasound, ophthalmologic evaluation, ECG (shortened QT interval).
  – Others: maternal endocrine status and family screening including molecular genetic studies

Management

• Acute
  – Expansion of extracellular fluid compartment and induced diuresis. Intravenous normal saline (10–20 ml/kg) with intravenous potent loop diuretic (furosemide 2 mg/kg). Reassess and repeat as needed.
    - monitor fluid balance and serum calcium (Ca), magnesium (Mg), sodium (Na), potassium (K) and osmolality q 6–8 hours. Prolonged diuresis may require Mg ± K replacement.
  – In neonates with low serum phosphorus (P) (<5 mg/dl), phosphate supplement of 0.5–1 mmol (15–30 mg) elemental P/kg/d in divided doses may normalize serum P and lower serum Ca.
  – Minimal data on the use of hormonal and other drug therapy.
• Maintenance
  – Depending on underlying cause
  – Low calcium, no vitamin D infant formula (Calcilo XD, Ross Products Division, Abbott Laboratories) may be needed
  – Minimal sunlight exposure to lower endogenous synthesis of vitamin D may be helpful
• Genetic counseling as appropriate

References

1. Bainbridge RR, Koo WWK, Tsang RC: Neonatal calcium and phosphorus disorders. In Lifshitz F (ed). *Pediatric Endocrinology: A Clinical Guide*. 3rd Ed. New York, Marcel Dekker Inc., 1996:473–496.

2. Mimouni F, Koo WWK. Neonatal mineral metabolism. In Tsang RC (ed). *Calcium and Magnesium Metabolism in Early Life*. Boca Raton, FL, CRC Press 1995:71–89.

9

Preterm Infants with Fractures

Winston Koo

Pathophysiology

- Low body store of bone nutrients at birth
- Inadequate nutrient intake, in particular calcium and phosphorus ± relative vitamin D deficiency
- Prolonged excessive pharmacotherapy, in particular, loop diuretic and corticosteroid
- Excessive force in physical restraint (e.g., during surgery) or in physical therapy
- Total parenteral nutrition in the presence of chronic cholestasis and unreplaced large volume intestinal secretory losses
- Familial conditions associated with bone disease

Clinical Features

- Incidence inversely related to birth weight and gestational age
- Chronologic age: usually <6 months, mostly at 2–4 months after birth
- Pattern of weight change: can occur during catch-up growth
- Dietary history: low calcium and low phosphorus intake
- Illness and medications: complicated postnatal course with multiple medications, in particular, loop diuretic and corticosteroid
- Initial presentation
  - Complications of fracture, e.g., immobilization or deformity
  - Incidental finding from x-rays taken for other purposes
  - Routine x-ray screening
- Physical examination
  - Anthropometric measurements at low percentile
  - Fracture-associated immobilization and deformity
  - Classic rachitic features
    - frequent but nonspecific, e.g., craniotabes and pot belly, since all small preterm infants have soft skulls and relatively large abdomens
    - infrequent, e.g., rachitic "rosary" of enlarged costochondral junction
    - rare, e.g., kyphoscoliosis and bowing because of absence of weight bearing at presentation

Diagnostic Work-up (Usual changes indicated as Normal, ↑ or ↓.)

- Radiographic skeletal survey: document extent of fractures and presence of rickets
- Serum biochemistry: Ca (N), Mg (N), P (↓), total alkaline phosphatase (N-↑), renal function tests (N) (creatinine, urea, electrolyte, bicarbonate), liver function tests, [total protein (N-↓), albumin (N-↓), Alanine aminotransferase (N-↑), bilirubin (N-↑)]
- Urine biochemistry: Ca (N↑), P (↓), creatinine (N)
- Vitamin D metabolites: 25 hydroxyvitamin D (N-↓), 1,25 dihydroxyvitamin D (N-↑)
- Others as necessary or investigational
  - Calciotropic hormones, e.g., parathyroid hormone (N-↑)
  - Bone turnover marker (N-↑): osteocalcin, bone specific alkaline phosphatase, C terminal propeptide of type I procollagen, C terminal telopeptide of type I collagen, pyridinoline, hydroxyproline
  - Dual energy x-ray absorptiometry (↓)

Treatment and Follow-up

- Minimize pain associated with fractures: splint ± analgesic
- Adequate overall nutritional support, in particular, high-mineral-containing parenteral nutrition and preterm infant formula
- Minimize pharmacotherapy that may affect bone mineralization
- Treat underlying disorders, e.g., liver disease, as necessary
- Serum and urine biochemistry q weekly until normal
- Radiographs q 1–3 months until normal healing and remodeling
- Other tests, if abnormal at baseline
- Follow-up until normal growth (serial anthropometric measurements plotted on growth chart) and development, resolution of deformity, and appropriate dietary intake (for age) is assured

References

1. Koo WWK, Steichen JJ: Osteopenia and Rickets of Prematurity. In Polin R, Fox W (eds). *Fetal and Neonatal Physiology*. 2nd Ed. Philadelphia, W.B. Saunders Company, 1998:2335–49.

2. Koo WWK. Laboratory assessment of nutritional metabolic bone disease in infants. *Clinical Biochemistry* 1996;29:429-438.

10

Rickets

Winston Koo

Pathophysiology

Undermineralization of cartilaginous epiphyseal growth plate during longitudinal growth, of cancellous bone during remodelling, and of periosteal bone during appositional growth.

Primarily Calcipenic

- Dietary deficiency (Small preterm infants received enteral or parenteral nutrients with low calcium and/or low phosphorus.)
- Vitamin D deficiency: ↓ intake or secondary to fat malabsorption, prolonged anticonvulsant therapy, renal failure, liver disease (?)
- Pseudodeficiency of vitamin D–vitamin-D-dependent rickets
  - Type I—classic 1α hydroxylase deficient: A/recessive
  - Type II—hypocalcemic vitamin-D-resistant rickets: hereditary defects in the interaction of calcitriol and its target tissues

Primarily Phosphopenic

- Dietary deficiency (Small preterm infants received enteral or parenteral nutrients with low calcium and/or low phosphorus.)
- Renal wasting
  - Familial hypophosphatemic rickets (X linked dom, A/ rec, X linked rec with hypercalciuria)
  - Renal tubular defect: primary or secondary to cystinosis, tyrosinemia, Wilson's disease, type I glycogen storage disease
- Other causes
  - McCune-Albright syndrome—more frequently present with hyperactivity of endocrine systems, e.g., precocious puberty, thyrotoxicosis, and acromegaly
  - Tumor or oncogenic—usually associated with benign, small mesenchymal tumor

The Bone and Mineral Manual
Copyright ©1999 by Academic Press
All rights of reproduction in any form reserved.

Clinical Manifestations

- Varies with age
- Failure to thrive, especially poor length gain
- Delayed fontanelle closure
- Classical rickets (nonspecific or uncommon in preterm infants—see chapter 9)
  - Frontal bossing, craniotabes, enlarged costochondral junction, wrists, ankles and knees
  - Kyphoscoliosis and bowing of legs—genu varum <3 to 4 years and genu valgum usually at school age
- Developmental delay with "regression" of motor function—the latter presumably in part secondary to bone pain.
- Delayed dentition or loss of existing teeth
- Extraskeletal manifestations
  - Hypocalcemic tetany and seizures in calcipenic rickets
  - Weakness and myopathy including protuberant abdomen from phosphate deficiency
- Features associated with specific underlying cause: e.g., alopecia associated with type II vitamin-D-dependent rickets

Radiographic Features

- Bone demineralization, cupping, fraying, and widening of the metaphyses
- Deformities of long bone associated with weight bearing
- Features of hyperparathyroidism may be present

Biochemical and Hormonal Changes in Calcipenic Rickets*

| | Serum | | | | | | | Urine | |
	Ca	P	AP	HCO_3	25 OHD	$1,25(OH)_2D$	PTH	Ca	P
Dietary deficiency	↓	N-↓	↑	N	N	↑-N	↑	↓	↑
Vitamin D deficiency	↓	↓	↑	N	↓	N-↑	↑	↓	↑
Pseudovitamin D deficiency									
Type I	↓	↓	↑	N	N	↓	↑	↓	↑
Type II	↓	↓	↑	N	N	↑	↑	↓	↑

*Usual changes depicted as N, ↑ or ↓

Biochemical and Hormonal Changes in Phosphopenic Rickets*

	Serum							Urine	
	Ca	P	AP	HCO$_3$	25 OHD	1,25(OH)$_2$D	PTH	Ca	P
Dietary deficiency	N	↓	↑	N	N	↑	N-↑	N-↑	↓
Renal Wasting									
Familial									
X dominant	N	↓	↑	N	N	N†	N-↑‡	N-↑‡	↑
A/recessive	N	↓	↑	N	N	↑	N	N	↑
X/recessive	N	↓	↑	N	N	↑	N	↑	↑
Renal tubular dysfunction	N	↓	↑	↓-N	N	↓-N	↑	↑	↑
Others:									
McCune-Albright	N	↓	↑	N	N	N	N	N	↑
Tumor	N	↓	↑	N	N	↓-N	N	N	↑

* Usual changes depicted as N, ↑ or ↓

† Normal range but inappropriately low for the extent of hypophosphatemia

‡ Hyperparathyroidism may be secondary to excessive P or inadequate 1,25(OH)$_2$D treatment. Hypercalciuria may be secondary to excessive 1,25(OH)$_2$D.

Management

- Aim to achieve normal growth and development
- Acute symptomatology, e.g., hypocalcemic tetany
- General dietary counseling—may need calcium and/or phosphate supplement
- Specific therapy varies with underlying disorder, e.g., physiologic doses of vitamin D for dietary vitamin D deficiency or 1,25(OH)$_2$D for Type I vitamin-D-dependent rickets. Greater doses of 1,25(OH)$_2$D are needed for type II vitamin-D-dependent rickets.
- Genetic counseling as appropriate
- Follow-up may be life-long depending on underlying cause.

References

1. Gertner JM. Rickets and disorders of vitamin D and phosphate metabolism. In Lifshitz F (ed). *Pediatric Endocrinology: A Clinical Guide.* 3rd Ed. New York, Marcel Dekker, Inc. 1996:507–519.

2. Glorieux FH. Rickets, the continuing challenge. *N Engl J Med* 1991; 325:1875–1877.

3. Koo WWK. Laboratory assessement of nutritional metabolic bone disease in infants. *Clin Biochem* 1996; 29:429–438.

4. Koo WWK, Steichen JJ: Osteopenia and rickets of prematurity. In Polin R, Fox W (eds), *Fetal and Neonatal Physiology*, 2nd Ed. Philadelphia, W.B. Saunders Company, 1998:2335–49.

5. Koo WWK, Tsang RC: Building better bones: calcium, magnesium, phosphorus, and vitamin D. In Tsang RC et al. (eds), *Nutrition During Infancy: Principles and Practice.* Philadelphia, Hanley and Belfus, Inc., 1997:175–207.

11

Osteogenesis Imperfecta

Jay R. Shapiro, Rebecca L. Slayton,
Paul Sponsellor

Definition

Osteogenesis imperfecta (OI) is a syndrome characterized by skeletal fragility as a result of several different mutations affecting the pro-α1 and pro-α2 chains of type I collagen. Type I collagen is the main structural protein of bone, skin, ligament and tendon. Frequently observed characteristics of OI include skeletal deformity, blue sclerae, adult onset hearing loss, scoliosis, joint laxity, and short stature. However OI is a heterogeneous disorder both clinically and genetically. Although in many patients the diagnosis of OI is clinically apparent, consideration must be given to other osteopenic syndromes in each age category.

The incidence of this condition is approximately 1:20,000 live births. An estimated 15,000 individuals in the United States have OI.

Table 1	Clinical Classification	Inheritance
Type 1	Mild OI; osseous fragility (variable from minimal through moderately severe), distinctly blue sclerae (at all ages); presenile hearing loss; limited skeletal deformity; mild short stature. Subgroup IA: with dentinogenesis imperfecta** Subgroup IB: no dentinogenesis imperfecta	AD
Type II	Lethal perinatal OI; extremely severe skeletal fragility with soft calvarium; micromelia; severe pulmonary insufficiency; stillbirth or neonatal death. Subgroup A: x-rays show broad crumpled long bones and broad ribs with continuous beading (fracture callus). Subgroup B: x-rays show broad crumpled long bones. Ribs show discontinuous beading or are not beaded. Subgroup C: x-rays show thin, fractured long bones and thin, beaded ribs.	AD

**Dentinogenesis imperfecta occurs in each clinical phentoype. The subgroup A and B can be applied to each category, however its value in subcategorization is uncertain.

| Type III: | Severe osseous fragility, usually congenital fractures, white or blue sclerae, variable but severe deformities of long bones, calvarial molding (tam o'shanter deformity) scoliosis with pectus wall deformity; basilar invagination; joint laxity; marked growth retardation with short stature; usually wheelchair bound. | AD/AR** |

           **True AR inheritance is rare compared to the probable frequency of parental mosaicism

| Type IV | Moderately severe OI with variable but clinically significant skeletal deformity and scoliosis; scleral color usually white, may be blue in childhood and may persist to adulthood; growth retardation is less marked than in type III; hearing loss; short stature (<5th percentile). | AD |

AD = autosomal dominant
AR = autosomal recessive

Differential Diagnosis

In the newborn
- Heritable chondrodystrophies
  - Thanatophoric dwarfism
  - Achondroplasia
- Congenital lethal hypophosphatasia

In children
- Childhood abuse
- Idiopathic juvenile osteoporosis
- Childhood hypophosphatasia
- Endocrinopathy-induced osteopenia: hyperthyroidism, glucocorticoid excess
- Malabsorption syndromes
- Lymphoma, leukemia

In adults
- Idiopathic familial osteoporosis
- Secondary causes of osteoporosis: endocrinopathy (hypogonadism; parathyroid adrenal and thyroid hormone excess)
- Adult (mild) hypophosphatasia
- Hypophosphataemic rickets
- Malabsorption

Secondary causes of osteoporosis in OI women and men
- Hyperthyroidism, hyperparathyroidism, glucocorticoid excess, hypogonadism, malabsorption syndromes, and malignancy.

Clinical Phenotypes

Type I
• Clinically mild disease, little or no skeletal deformity
• Parents may be affected or spontaneous occurrence.
• Height is usually reduced for age but may be normal in a few individuals.
• Sclerae are always blue.
• Fractures may or may not be present at birth: the first fracture can occur at any age and may be delayed until the second decade.
• Fractures typically heal with little deformity.
• Mild joint laxity.
• Vertebral deformities due to endplate fracture
• Scoliosis is mild and tends not to progress with increasing age.
• Adult onset hearing loss occurs in the second to third decade.

Type II   (*see Table 1 for radiologic classification*)
• Infants have shortened deformed limbs, but body length may be normal.
• Associated with perinatal death in the majority
• Pulmonary insufficiency is responsible in the majority.
• Intracranial bleeding due to birth trauma may occur.
• Thoracic wall injury with muscular weakness may lead to mechanical respiratory insufficiency.
• Pulmonary hypoplasia may occur.
• Occasionally an infant with this phenotype may survive for a variable period in the setting of intensive medical care.

Type III
• Skeletal demineralization is severe: subjects are wheelchair bound.
• Fractures with deformities are present at birth.
• Wormian bones in the occipital calvarium present at birth: may persist through the first decade.
• Sclerae are white in many type III cases: blue sclerae may be present.
• Dentinogenesis imperfecta occurs in approximately 20%.
• Cranial molding is common with a palpable occipital overhang presenting the "helmet" or "tam o'shanter" deformity.
• Molding of the forehead causes a characteristic "sunset" appearance of facies due to apparent lowering of the cornea with exposed blue sclerae above.
• There is marked growth retardation: individuals are approximately 36 inches in height as adults.
• Deformity of the lower extremities is usually more severe than that of the upper extremities: deformity of the humerus and radius/ulna occurs and may require surgical correction.
• Joint laxity of a moderate extent
• Fractures of both the long bones and vertebrae occur.
• Progressive thoracic deformity may lead to cardiac insufficiency.

Type IV
- This phenotype is intermediate in severity between type I (mild) and type III (severe).
- Characterized by decrease in stature, scoliosis, and moderately severe skeletal deformities that may require mechanical assistance to ambulation.
- Sclerae typically are blue in childhood and lighten in adults.
- Radiologically, there may be an advanced degree of skeletal dysplasia, bony deformity, and osteoporosis.
- Cane or wheelchair is required for ambulation.

Associated Phenotypes
- OI associated with joint contractures (Bruck syndrome)
- OI associated with renal calculi
- Unusual complication of chronic renal failure due to obstructive uropathy secondary to bony pelvic outlet deformity

Other Clinical Characteristics and Complications

Ocular Complications
- Corneal and scleral collagen fibers are diminished in diameter.
- The scleral coat may be thinned.
- Scleral rupture
- Keratoconus

Dentinogenesis Imperfecta (DI)
- The teeth have a brown translucent appearance and rapidly wear down.
- Occurs in each phenotype; rare in fluid type I disease, more common in type II/IV
- May affect 20–75% of individuals with type III/IV disease
- Decidious teeth are more severely affected than permanent teeth.
- The penetrance of this trait is very high for affected members of a family.
- Multiple radiolucent mandibular cysts have been reported in certain families.

Hearing Loss
- Damage to the stapes crura occurs early in life.
- Sensorineural and conductive hearing loss occur, more commonly in type I disease.
- Onset occurs during the second or third decade and is progressive with age. Stapedectomy may be effective.

Cardiopulmonary Disease
- Clinically significant cardiac disease is uncommon.
- In children and adults with type Ill disease, cardiac failure may occur secondary to restrictive pulmonary insufficiency.
- Aortic regurgitation with annuloaortic ectasia
- Mitral regurgitation
- Mitral valve prolapse is present in approximately 8%.
- Pulmonary insufficiency occurs in type II disease at birth.
- Pulmonary hypoplasia may occur due to inadequate bronchoalveolar development.

Basilar Invagination
- More likely to occur in type III disease
- Symptoms include chronic headache, lower cranial nerve dysfunction, distal limb paresthesiae, hyperreflexia, clonus and spasticity, and nystagmus
- Brainstem compression with respiratory compromise and hydrocephalus may occur.
- Posterior fossa decompression and occipito-cervical fusion may be required.
- Basilar invagination tends to progress in severe OI.

Hypercalciuria and renal calculi
- Primary hypercalciuria has been reported to affect approximately 25% of OI children
- Not associated with the formation of renal calculi: renal calculi have been observed in OI children shortly after birth or at older ages. This is not associated with hypercalciuria.
- Transient renal papillary calcification has also been observed.
- Consider renal calculi in children with signs of infection or hematuria

Hyperplastic Callus
- An uncommon complication; occurs during fracture healing
- Appears as an inflammatory tumor-like mass at the fracture site
- May contain irregular calcification simulating osteosarcoma
- Treatment with anti-inflammatory agents is indicated.

Genetics

Summary of Collagen Mutations

In excess of 200 different mutations affecting either the pro-αl or pro-α2 chains of type I collagen have been reported in all OI phenotypes. In only a few cases have the mutations been identical. The helical portion of the type I collagen molecule is composed of the repeating triplet (Gly-X-Y). The majority of mutations are point mutations affecting the collagen triple helix with a cysteine substitution for the first-position glycine (Gly) being the most common. Other point substitutions for glycine include serine, valine, aspartate and argenine. However, insertions and deletions of varying sizes have been reported in each phenotype. In type I OI (mild) these may lead to premature termination codons with degradation of the mutant mRNA in the nucleus. The effect is to decrease collagen production by one-half; however, the collagen secreted into extracellular matrix is normally assembled. In types II, III, and IV, the mutant alpha chain is assembled and secreted into the extracellular matrix producing structurally abnormal bone. Mutations located at N-terminal positions tend to be clinically mild. Those at the C-terminus, from which folding of the alpha chains proceed, tend to be more severe. However, exceptions to this have been observed, so that there is no strict relationship between the type of mutation and its location, and the clinical phenotype.

Inheritance as a Dominant Trait

The majority of OI cases in each phenotype are the result of structural type I collagen mutations and are therefore transmitted in a dominant manner.

Inheritance as a Recessive Trait

Most OI cases are the result of structural collagen mutations and are inherited as dominants. The empiric recurrence rate for severe OI (III) approximates 6-7 %. The frequency of true recessive inheritance in type III disease is probably less than 1%. Recurrent cases previously considered recessive are now recognized as the result of gonadal mosaicism.

Mosaicism

Gonadal mosaicism is now recognized as responsible for the majority of type II or type III cases that were attributed to recessive inheritance. Parents of both sporadic and recurrent type III/IV cases should be carefully examined for subtle signs of OI including decreased bone mineral density, short stature, and joint laxity.

Clinical Diagnosis

Prenatal Diagnosis

Where a specific type I mutation has been identified in a proband, the occurrence of OI may be defined by chorionic villus biopsy during the first trimester or ultrasound during the second trimester. Ultrasound may not disclose OI in mild disease.

X-ray *(See Table I)*

Diminished bone mass is present in most OI subjects except in mild disease (type I) where cortical thickness may approximate normal. Vertebral compression fractures may occur. In severe disease, the shaft of long bones appears thin and the epiphyseal region may appear bulbous, with indistinct epiphyses. In severe disease, the epiphyseal region contains calcified whorls of matrix ("popcorn" sign).

Bone Mineral Density

DXA bone mineral determination may be technically difficult in certain OI subjects because of scoliosis and skeletal deformities. Bone mineral density is decreased in almost all patients with OI. Infrequently in type I disease, adult bone mineral density approaches normal values for age and gender.

Biomarkers of Bone Turnover

Serum biomarkers osteocalcin, alkaline phosphatase, and procollagen peptides (N-terminal and C-terminal propeptides). The majority of patients have normal to low values suggesting low bone turnover. Serum procollagen peptides reflecting collagen synthesis by osteoblasts have been consistently reported as depressed in OI patients. The urinary excretion of collagen crosslinks (pyridinoline crosslinks, N-telopeptide excretion, and C-terminal crosslink excretion) as indicators of collagen resorption are normal to low in many subjects, but they are elevated in about 15% of patients suggesting elevated bone turnover in those individuals.

Molecular and Biochemical Diagnosis

A 4–6 mm dermal biopsy provides fibroblast cells for the study of collagen metabolism, as well as the recovery of DNA and RNA for gene analysis. A skin biopsy obtained from a patient is grown in culture for 4 to 6 weeks. At this time, the cultured fibroblast cells can be used for collagen studies and can provide DNA and RNA for molecular analysis. White blood cells can also be harvested to provide DNA for molecular analysis.

Type I

Decreased production of the pro-α1 chain due to decreased steady-state levels of COL1A1 mRNA in the nucleus.
- Biochemical Analysis
  - Evaluation of quantity of pro-α1 (I): [^{3}H]proline-labeled procollagens are harvested and separated in SDS-polyacrylamide gels. In cells from type I patients, the ratio of pro-α1 (I) to pro-α1 (III) is decreased (1:1) compared with normal (3:1).
- Molecular Analysis
  - To confirm that the reduction in the pro-α1 (I) chain is a result of decreased steady-state levels of COL1A1 mRNA, mRNA from each allele is labeled with ^{32}P-dATP separated by restriction endonuclease digestion at a polymorphic site (Mnl I) located downstream of the translation termination signal. This method is limited by the fact that not all individuals are heeterozygous at this site.

Types II–IV

Structurally abnormal α1 or α2 chain usually due to glycine substitution, overmodification of collagen chains is common that alters chain migration in SDS-gels.
- Biochemical Analysis
  - Evaluation of overmodification of type I chains: [^{3}H]proline-labeled procollagen chains are partially pepsin lysed to remove the N-and C-terminal propeptides prior to electrophoresis. Overmodification is seen as a shift in the peptide band relative to samples from normal individuals.
- Molecular Analysis
  - In heterogenous individuals, levels of mRNA from each allele should be equal.

Mutation Detection

Although not done frequently and usually as a research tool, collagen gene sequence may be determined for the purpose of diagnosis. Genomic DNA is isolated from serum or cells and the two genes for type I collagen (COL1A1 and COL1A2) are screened by polymerase chain reaction (PCR) followed by single strand conformation polymorphism (SSCP) gel electrophoresis, conformation sensitive gel electrophoresis (CSGE), or one of the many other techniques that detects sequence variations in a sample.

Interpretation of Results

Although the diagnosis of OI can often be made based on clinical findings, in some cases it may not be as clear. The results of a skin biopsy can help differentiate between type I OI and mild forms of type IV OI or between other disorders that would be included in the differential diagnosis.

Bone Biopsies in Diagnosis

- Iliac crest bone biopsies are usually not required for diagnosis in OI.
- Tetracycline double-labeling prior to biopsy is required for histomorphometric analysis.
- Indications
  - Osteomalacia secondary to malabsorption, drugs
  - Coexistent cancer
- Characteristics
  - Decreased bone volume
  - Apparent increase in number of osteocytes
  - Decreased trabecular thickness
  - Decreased cortical thickness
  - Decreased mineral apposition rate

Medical Treatment

- There is no confirmed medical therapy.
- Assure adequate calcium and vitamin D intake; because of hypercalcemia reported in approximately 30%, measure urinary calcium excretion before increasing diet calcium.
- Estrogen/progesterone replacement is advisable in postmenopausal women.
- Testosterone replacement is appropriate for men with low serum-free testosterone.
- *Bisphosphonates*: Initial data based on bone biopsy after one year of treatment in children with types III and IV OI, and two years of treatment in adults with type I OI indicates that the second generation bisphosphonate, pamidronate, may retard bone loss.
- *Fluoride*: A single trial of fluoride therapy in OI conducted in a mixed population of children did not disclose a change in bone histomorphometry or mineral densitometry. Administered as sodium fluoride in a dose of 1 mg/kg/day. (M Whyte, Washington University, St. Louis)
- *Growth Hormone*: A clinical trial of growth hormone at the National Institutes of Health (National Institute Child Health and Development) suggests that type IV OI may show an increase in height above expected. No effect of growth hormone administration was seen in other OI phenotypes.

Orthopedic Approach

- Continuous orthopedic care is essential for minimizing deformity and maximizing function. Skeletal loading is effective in building bone mass and although its effect in OI is not yet investigated, there seems to be benefit. Therefore, mobility is encouraged through the use of
  - Foam mold casting and supportive bracing
  - Physical therapy
  - Internal fixation
- Intramedullary stabilization is beneficial for two categories of patients.
  - Those with progressive bowing that impairs use of the extremities
  - Those experiencing repeated multiple fractures
- Rods inside bone are more effective than plates.
  - The Bailey-Dubrow rod is expandable as children grow.
  - Steinman pins are useful in infants.
- Limb length inequality or angular deformities
  - Correct at or near the end of growth
  - Ilizarov device for external fixation if bone is mildly brittle
  - Osteotomy and implanted rods for severe skeletal fragility
- Spinal deformity occurs in the majority of severe OI patients.
  - If over 80–100 degrees, it will contribute to pulmonary insufficiency
  - Bracing is not effective.
  - A curve over 40 degrees is likely to progress.
    - surgery recommended for curves over 40-50 degrees if OI is not severe
    - correction and stabilization with rods anchored in every vertebra usually necessary
  - Progression to severity should not be allowed because correction is not possible to the extent seen with idiopathic scoliosis.
  - Spinal surgery may be futile with markedly defective bone matrix.
- Basilar invagination
  - Bracing may help if a brace from chin to trunk is tolerated.
  - Posterior fusion from skull to upper cervical spine
  - Decompression for signs of neurologic compression involving anterior transoral removal of odontoid, anterior arch of C1 and possibly the clivus. Plate fixation and fusion in the back provides support for the neck.
- Treatment of fractures with surgery or casting
  - Treat with cast if mobility is not impaired.
  - If severe OI precludes effective fixation, cast or brace may be preferable.
  - If cast restricts mobility, surgery is advisable.
  - Surgery if fracture is difficult to control in a cast

Rehabilitation Therapy

- Periodic functional assessment and ongoing rehabilitative care are important.
  - Assess motor skills.
  - Strength assessment
  - Joint range of motion
    - hyperextensibility
    - contractures
  - Gait analysis
  - Neurologic assessment
  - Orthotic devices for joint laxity
  - Lower extremity bracing in polypropylene braces to facilitate ambulation.
  - Water aerobic conditioning programs are very useful in maintaining muscle mass and strength.
- Therapy to restore joint motion and muscle strength is important following fractures, particularly if casting or surgery has ensued.

References

1. Avioli L, Krane SM (eds). *Osteogenesis Imperfecta in Metabolic Bone Disease.* 3rd Ed. Philadelphia: WB Saunders, 1997.

2. Lund AM, Nicholls AC, Skorby F. Parental mosaicism and autosomal dominant mutations causing structural abnormalities of collagen I are frequent in families with osteogenesis imperfecta type III/IV. *Acta Paediatr* 1997;86: 711–71.

3. Pepin M, Atkinson M, Starman B, Byers PH. Strategies and outcomes of prenatal diagnosis for osteogenesis imperfecta: A review of biochemical and molecular studies completed in 129 pregnancies. *Prenatal Diagnosis* 1997; 17: 559–570.

4. Smith R, Francis MJO, Houghton, GR. *The Brittle Bone Syndrome: Osteogenesis Imperfecta.* London: Butterworths, 1983.

12

Juvenile Osteoporosis

Jorge A. Prada
Reginald C. Tsang

Definition

- A primary osteoporosis that develops at the time of the pubertal growth spurt
- A dissociation between linear growth and consolidation of the skeleton

Clinical Features

- Onset between ages 8–14
- Abrupt onset of bone pain, spinal deformity, fragility fractures
- Vertebral fractures (cause of pain) mainly lower thoracic upper lumbar
- May be self-limited but patient is left with long-term consequences of deformities

Radiology

- Skeletal demineralization without features of rickets or excessive bone resorption
- Vertebral fractures usually affect anterior height but may have "codfish" appearance.
- BMD by densitometry is low.

Laboratory

- Usually normal serum chemistry
- Occasionally increased calcium, decreased PTH
- Urine calcium and markers of bone resorption may be increased.

Differential Diagnosis

- Osteogenesis imperfecta
  - Family history is absent in osteoporosis
  - Different radiologic features
- Secondary osteoporosis
  - Same causes as in adults, but all are rare

The Bone and Mineral Manual
Copyright ©1999 by Academic Press

Therapy

- Supportive care
- Non-weight-bearing crutch walking
- Pharmacologic (none well documented to be helpful because condition is too uncommon to complete formal clinical trials)
  - Calcium   500–1000 mg/day
  - Calcitonin   200 units intranasally/day
                     50 units sc three times per week
  - Calcitriol   0.25–0.5 mcg/day
  - Phosphate   0.5 g orally, tid

13

Fibrous Dysplasia

Frederick S. Kaplan

Fibrous Dysplasia

- Fibrous dysplasia is a sporadic skeletal disorder caused by somatic activating mutations in the gene for the alpha subunit of the stimulatory G-protein of adenylyl cyclase. The disorder causes focal expansion of one or more bones due to the developmental arrest of normal osteogenesis and the pathologic development of osteogenic fibrous tissue within the bone marrow space. Fibrous dysplasia leads to skeleton deformity, pain and pathologic fractures.
- Usually diagnosed in children in the first decade of life on the basis of bone pain, deformity, pathologic fracture, headache or cranial neuropathy
- A prominent cause of morbidity but not mortality
- Monostotic, polyostotic, or associated focal hyperpigmentation of skin (café-au-lait), endocrinopathies, growth disturbance, precocious puberty (McCune-Albright syndrome)

Most Common Symptoms

- Bone pain
- Skeletal deformity
- Pathologic fracture

Radiographic Appearance

- Unicameral or multicameral expansile radiolucent lesions ("ground-glass")
- Lesions may be in metaphysis or diaphysis
- Lesions cause focal osteoporosis of the cortex of the bone with a scalloped appearance of the endosteal surface

Histologic Appearance

- Primitive-appearing chaotic whirls of fibrous stroma
- Arrested osteogenesis with woven-bone and ill-defined irregular-shaped trabecula ("Chinese letters" appearance) arising directly out of the fibrous stroma.

Skeletal Complications

- Pathologic fracture with normal healing of the subperiosteal bone and abnormal healing of endosteal bone
- Skeletal deformity due to focal proliferation of fibrous tissue in marrow cavity and imperfect osteogenesis; may cause visual disturbances, headaches and other cranial neuropathies if the skull is involved
- Limb-length discrepancy with limp
- Bone pain
- Rarely undergoes malignant degeneration

Indications for Surgery

- To limit progressive deformity
- To treat nonunion of fractures and facilitate fracture healing
- To relieve intractable bone pain
- To improve mobility
- To relieve focal pressure on affected nerves

Surgical Procedures

- Curettage of affected bone followed by grafting with normal autologous bone or with banked bone; bone affected with fibrous dysplasia should not be used for bone graft
- Prophylactic rodding of long bone with impending pathologic fractures
- Corrective osteotomies with internal fixation and bone grafting

Medical Treatment

- Increased bone resorption at the periphery of fibrous dysplasia lesions suggests that anti-resorptive medications may be helpful in controlling disease symptoms and limiting disease activity.
- Intermittent treatment with cyclical intravenous pamidronate have been effective in some patients and can alleviate bone pain through a reduction of bone turnover.
- The aromatase inhibitor, testolactone, may be used to decrease estrogen levels in females with precocious puberty and the McCune-Albright syndrome.

McCune–Albright Syndrome (1937)

- Polyostotic fibrous dysplasia (often unilateral)
- Multiple café-au-lait lesions (coast of Maine)
- Precocious puberty
- Other endocrine hyperactivity
- Not genetically inherited in the Mendelian manner
- Postzygotic somatic-activating mutations in the alpha subunit of the stimulatory G-protein of adenylyl cyclase (GNAS-1)

- Localized increased production of cAMP in somatic tissues leads to increased activation of the cAMP responsive element in the cFos gene in those cells.
- Sustained elevations of the Fos protein in target tissues of skin, bone and endocrine organs leads to the disease phenotype.
- Similar molecular findings are also found with more restricted disease activity in isolated monostotic and polyostotic fibrous dysplasia without skin or endocrine manifestations.

Endocrine Overactivity that May Be Associated with McCune-Albright Syndrome

- Precocious puberty
- Hyperthyroidism
- Hyperparathyroidism
- Acromegaly
- Cushing's disease

References

1. Candeliere GA, Glorieux FH, Prud'homme J, St.-Arnaud R. Increased expression of the c-fos proto-oncogene in bone from patients with fibrous dysplsia. *N Engl J Med* 1995; 332:1546–1551.

2. Chapurlat RD, Delmas PD, Liens D, Meunier PJ. Long-term effects of intravenous pamidronate in fibrous dysplasia of bone. *J Bone Mineral Res* 1997; 12:1746–1752.

3. Edgerton MT, Persing JA, Jane JA. The surgical treatment of fibrous dysplasia. With emphasis on recent contributions from cranio-maxillofacial surgery. *Ann Surg* 1985; 202:459–479.

4. Levine MA. The McCune-Albright Syndrome: The whys and wherefores of abnormal signal transduction. *N Engl J Med* 1991; 325:1738–1740.

5. Liens D, Delmas PD, Meunier PJ. Long-term effects of intravenous pamidronate in fibrous dysplasia of bone. *Lancet* 1994; 343:953–954.

6. Shenker A, Weinstein LS, Moran, et al. Severe endocrine and nonendocrine manifestations of the McCune-Albright syndrome associated with activating mutations of stimulating G protein GS-alpha. *J Pediatrics* 1993; 123:509–518.

7. Stanton RP, Montgomery BE. Fibrous dysplasia (review). *Orthopaedics* 1996; 19:679–685.

8. Stephenson RB, London MD, Hankin FM, Kaufer H. Fibrous dysplasia—an analysis of options for treatment. *J Bone Joint Surg* 1987; 69A:400–409.

9. Weinstein LS, Shenker A, Gejman PV, et al. Activating mutations of the stimulatory G protein in the McCune-Albright Syndrome. *N Engl J Med.* 1991; 325:1688–1695.

10. *Questions & Answers about Fibrous Dysplasia.* New York: The Paget Foundation, 1995.

14

Secondary Amenorrhea

Karen K. Miller
Anne Klibanski

Etiologies

- Hypothalamic amenorrhea—35%
- Polycystic ovarian syndrome—30%
- Hyperprolactinemia—15 to 20%
- Premature ovarian failure—10%
- Asherman's syndrome—7%
- Hypothyroidism—1%
- Cushing's syndrome—<1%

Causes Associated with Bone Loss

- Hypothalamic amenorrhea, including anorexia nervosa and increased exercise
- Premature ovarian failure
- Hyperprolactinemia
- Cushing's syndrome

Degree of Bone Loss

- The most severe bone loss is seen in women with anorexia nervosa. Fifty percent have bone densities more than 2 standard deviations below the means for their ages, and clinical fractures occur.
- Patients with hyperprolactinemia typically have up to a 20% loss of bone density, but clinical fractures are rare.
- Preferential trabecular bone loss is seen in estrogen deficiency.

The Bone and Mineral Manual
Copyright ©1999 by Academic Press
All rights of reproduction in any form reserved.

Evaluation

- **History:** Galactorrhea? Hot flashes? Anorexia nervosa? Excessive exercise? Stress? Symptoms of hypothyroidism? Hirsutism, acne or obesity? Sexually active? Instrumentation of the uterus?
- **Physical examination:** Abnormally thin or obese? Signs of androgen excess? Galactorrhea?
- Beta-HCG
- Prolactin
- TSH
- FSH
- Estradiol
- For osteopenic patients, exclude other causes of osteoporosis such as hyperparathyroidism, medication use, systemic illness, and vitamin D deficiency.

Therapy for Bone Loss

- Reversal of underlying condition (dopamine agonists in hyperprolactinemia, weight gain and psychological recovery in anorexia nervosa, decreased stress or exercise in hypothalamic amenorrhea, surgery to cure Cushing's syndrome)
- Estrogen (important in several states including premature ovarian failure but not proven effective in anorexia nervosa)
- Role of bisphosphonates not established

15

Nephrolithiasis

Murray J. Favus

Composition and Frequency of Kidney Stones

- Calcium oxalate in 15–30% of all stones.
- Ca oxalate may be either monohydrate (dumbbell-shaped) or dihydrate (bipyramidal).
- Ca P (elongated, narrow) may occur alone (5–15% of Ca stones) or more commonly, with Ca oxalate (30–45% of Ca stones).
- Infection stones (20% of all stones) are composed of struvite (magnesium ammonium phosphate) and are rectangular prisms.
- Uric acid stones (2–10% of all stones) are flat, rhomboidal-shaped.
- Cystine stones (1–3% of all stones) are hexagonal plates.

Clinical Manifestations of Stones by Stone Composition

- Spontaneous stone passage occurs with Ca, uric acid and cystine but rarely struvite.
- Small, separate stones suggest Ca and uric acid and occasionally cystine, not struvite.
- On x-ray, Ca and struvite are radio-dense while cystine is less dense.
- Uric acid stones are lucent and appear as a filling defect on IVP.
- Staghorn stones fill renal pelvis and may be struvite, uric acid, or cystine.
- Formation of sludge with obstruction occurs with either uric acid or cystine stones.

Active Stone Disease

- Adults with recurrent stones, multiple new stones within one year, or growing stones
- All children with kidney stones.

Diagnostic Evaluation of Stone-Formers

- Every effort should be made to identify the composition of each stone.
- All patients should have a plain radiograph of the abdomen and an IVP.
- Microscopic inspection of a freshly voided urine for cystalluria
- Note radiographic changes (lucent, opaque) and shape of crystals in urine (see the preceding section on stone composition).

Laboratory Evaluation of Stone-Formers

After the First Stone

- Needs only a basic evaluation if only one stone is formed
- Urinalysis
- Urine culture if infection is considered
- Blood calcium, phosphate, uric acid, creatinine
- Urine aliquot for cystine

Active Stone Disease

- Medication that may interfere with Ca or uric acid metabolism discontinued for at least 10–14 days (vitamin D, vitamin C, multivitamins, diuretics, Ca supplements, steroids, and acetazolamide [Diamox]) .
- 24-hour urine collection for volume, pH, concentration of Ca, phosphate, uric acid, sodium, oxalate, citrate, and creatinine
- Urine collection while patients eat their usual diet
- Fasting blood sample for calcium, phosphate, uric acid, creatinine

Pathogenesis of Stone

- Urine supersaturation with respect to stone crystals. May occur by increasing urine excretion, decreasing urine volume, or reduction in other ligands such as citrate that normally forms soluble Ca complexes rather than permitting formation of an insoluble complex of Ca oxalate
- Urine pH important in supersaturation of CaP (high urine pH favors crystal formation) and uric acid (low pH favors insoluble uric acid crystals), but not Ca oxalate
- Nucleation of crystals may occur in supersaturated urine with binding of crystals onto the surface of preformed crystals or particles in urine.
- Urine inhibitors of crystal growth such as citrate, pyrophosphate and proteins (uropontin, Tamm-Horsfall protein, nephrocalcin) reduce supersaturation, nucleation, adsorption, or crystal growth. Their absence (example: low urine citrate) may promote stone formation.

Causes of Ca Oxalate Stones

- Hypercalciuria
- Low urine citrate
- Hyperoxaluria
- Hyperuricosuria

Causes of Hypercalciuric Ca Oxalate Stone Formation*

- Definition of hypercalciuria. 24-hour urine >250 mg for women; >300 mg for men; or >4 mg/Kg body weight either sex; >140 mg/g urine creatinine
- Hypercalciuria with hypercalcemia
  - Primary hyperparathyroidism
  - Granulomatous disease

- Vitamin D intoxication
- Sarcoidosis
- Lithium carbonate
· Hypercalciuria with normocalcemia
  - Idiopathic (familial)
  - Sarcoidosis
  - Renal tubular acidosis
  - Hyperthyroidism
  - Immobilization
  - Paget's disease of bone
  - Rapidly progressive osteoporosis

* Adapted from Coe FL, Parks JH. Clinical Approach. In: *Nephrolithiasis: Pathogenesis and Treatment*, 2nd Edition, St. Louis: Mosby, pp. 1–37, 1988.

Causes of Low Urine Citrate (less than 500 mg/24 hour)

· Systemic acidosis
  - Renal tubular acidosis
  - Chronic diarrheal states
  - Ileostomy
· Thiazide-induced hypokalemia
· Urinary tract infection
· Idiopathic
· Glucocorticoid excess

Causes of Hyperoxaluria (24-hour urine oxalate greater than 45 mg)*

· Metabolic overproduction
  - Hereditary types I and II
  - Ethylene glycol ingestion
  - Methoxyflurane anesthesia
· Gastrointestinal overabsorption
  - Ileal resection
  - Small bowel bypass surgery
  - Pancreatic insufficiency
  - Celiac sprue
  - Selected dietary overingestion
  - Cellulose phosphate or low Ca diet

*Adapted from Klugman V, Favus MJ Diagnosis and treatment of calcium kidney stones. In: *Advances in Endocrinology and Metabolism*, EL Mazzaferri, RS Barr, RA Kreisberg, (Eds.). St. Louis: Mosby, pp.117–142, 1995.

Causes of Hyperuricosuria (24-hour urine uric acid >800 mg in men; >750 mg in women)

- Increased purine ingestion (meat, fish, poultry)
- Overproduction of uric acid
- Low urine pH
- Dehydration with low urine volumes and low urine pH

Pathogenesis of Idiopathic Hypercalciuria (IH)

- Familial, with evidence of genetic basis consistent with autosomal dominant inheritance
- Hypercalciuria is persistent with same frequency in children as adults (about 5–10% of general population).
- Stones are Ca oxalate alone or with minor amount of CaP with occasionally, uric acid crystals.
- Serum Ca is always normal. Parathyroid hormone is usually normal, and elevated in 5% of patients.
- Intestinal Ca hyperabsorption found in most patients
- Source of excess urine Ca is intestinal hyperabsorption when Ca intake is normal. When Ca intake is low, urine Ca may decrease to low levels (like non-stone formers), or may remain excessive (excessive urine Ca from bone resorption).
- Patients who do not conserve urine Ca during low Ca diet develop negative Ca balance. Serum 1,25-dihydroxyvitamin D_3 [1,25$(OH)_2D_3$] levels may be normal (22–56 pg/ml) or elevated during normal Ca intake.
- Bone mineral density is reduced in men and women.

Three Models of Hypercalciuria in IH

- All models have normal serum Ca and increased intestinal Ca absorption.
- Primary intestinal overabsorption
  - Normal serum 1,25$(OH)_2D_3$ and PTH
  - Maintain Ca balance during low Ca diet
- Primary overproduction of 1,25$(OH)_2D_3$
  - May have fasting hypercalciuria
  - Elevated serum 1,25$(OH)_2D_3$ and normal PTH
  - Negative Ca balance during low Ca diet
- Renal hypercalciuria
  - Fasting hypercalciuria
  - Elevated PTH and 1,25$(OH)_2D_3$
  - Intestinal Ca hyperabsorption secondary to increased 1,25$(OH)_2D_3$
  - Negative Ca balance during low Ca diet

Treatment of IH to Prevent Stones

- Reduce 24-hour urine Ca to 200 mg or below using a thiazide diuretic.
  - Chlorthalidone or indapamide once daily or hydrochlorothiazide twice daily
- Monitor serum K and replace if low using KCl, K citrate or Urocit-K.

- If urine citrate is also low, add potassium citrate or K-citrate-acetate-bicarbonate (Urocit-K) with each meal.
- Adequate hydration to maintain urine output of 1.5 liters daily
- Avoid dehydration
- Measurement of 24-hour urine Ca excretion 6–8 weeks after initiating therapy and yearly
- Dietary Ca restriction does not reduce stone recurrence and may create negative Ca balance and low bone density.
- Maintain adequate Ca diet of about 800 mg per day
- If 24-hour urine Ca remains above 200 mg/24-hour, then evaluate dietary Ca intake, compliance with medication, increase dose of thiazide, measure urine sodium excretion, and limit sodium intake if excessive.

Treatment of Hyperoxaluric States

- Enteric hyperoxalurias
  - Increased colon oxalate absorption due to a variety of factors may reach 100 mg/24 hr
- Decrease colon oxalate absorption
  - Low fat diet
  - Low oxalate diet
  - Oral Ca carbonate 250–1,000 mg with each meal to bind dietary oxalate
  - Cholestyramine resin 4–16 g/day in divided doses to bind luminal oxalate, and fatty acids and bile salts which increase colon permeability to oxalate
  - Oral citrate to bind and solubilize urine Ca
- Treat genetic hyperoxaluric states I and II.
  - Pyridoxine 400 mg/day
  - Urine volume of 3 L/day
  - Oral citrate
  - Combined liver and renal transplantation before systemic oxalosis develops
- Dietary hyperoxaluria from excessive consumption of foods high in oxalate
  - Oxalate-rich foods are spinach, rhubarb, parsley, pepper, nuts, chocolate, cocoa, and tea
  - Limit intake of oxalate-rich foods

Treatment of Hyperuricosuric Ca Oxalate Stone Formation

- Dietary overingestion of purine-rich foods is major source of urine uric acid.
- Overproduction of uric acid in minority of patients
- Avoid dehydration
- Maintain urine pH above 6.0 to improve uric acid solubility.
- Allopurinol 200 mg/day when hyperurocosuria is due to uric acid overproduction
- Allopurinol reduces new Ca oxalate stone formation and growth of preexisting stones.

Stone Removal

- Surgical removal of stones if they cause obstruction, severe pain, bleeding, serious infection
- Stones <5 mm may be passed spontaneously; > 7 mm tend not to pass
- Extracorporeal shock wave lithotripsy (ESWL) indicated for:
  - Stones less than 2 cm
  - Presence of a single stone in renal parenchyma
  - Location in upper two-thirds of ureter
- Other procedures
  - Ureterolithotomy for stones >2 cm; stones in lower one-third of ureter; large infected stones; stones in the ureteropelvic junction or in calyceal diverticulae

Suggested Readings

1. Coe FL, MJ Favus, CYC Pak, JH Parks, and GM Premminger (eds.). *Kidney Stones: Medical and Surgical Management.* Philadelphia: Lippincott-Raven Publishers, 1996.

2. Coe FL, and JH Parks. Nephrolithiasis. In: Favus MJ (ed.). *Primer on the Metabolic Bone Diseases and Disorders of Mineral Metabolism.* 3rd Edition. Philadelphia; Lippincott-Raven Press, pp. 433–437.

3. Lemann J Jr. Pathogenesis of idiopathic hypercalciuria In: Coe FL and MJ Favus (eds.). *Disorders of Bone and Mineral Metabolism.* New York: Raven Press, 1992; pp. 685–706.

4. Monk RD, and DA Bushinsky. Pathogenesis of idiopathic hypercalciuria In: Coe FL, Favus MJ, Pak CYC, Parks JH, and GM Premminger (eds.). *Kidney Stones: Medical and Surgical Management.* Philadelphia: Lippincott-Raven Publishers, 1996; pp. 759–772.

16

Acute Spinal Cord Injury, Closed Head Injury, and Reflex Sympathetic Dystrophy

Albert C. Clairmont
Velimir Matkovic

Acute Spinal Cord Injury

Definition

- Acute spinal cord injury (SCI) is characterized by sustained damage to neural elements in the spinal canal, resulting in impairment or loss of motor and or sensory function. This is described as quadriplegia if the cervical segments are involved and paraplegia if thoracic, lumbar, or sacral segments are involved.

Epidemiology

- Incidence rate in the United States is 30 to 40 cases per million population. Prevalence in the United States is between 183,000 and 230,000 people.

Causes

- Motor vehicle accidents—44.5%
- Falls—18.1%
- Acts of violence—16.6%
- Sports—12.7%
- Other—8.1%

Complications at Bone Tissue Level

Disuse Osteoporosis

- Increased bone resorption, decreased bone formation
- Rapid bone loss primarily in the paralyzed limbs (22% in distal femur in the first three months; 27% at four months; 40–45% in pelvic bones after one year; lower limb bone loss of 25% at the end of first year; and long-term bone loss of 50%) (Figure 1).
- Biochemical markers of bone resorption increased, peaks ~6 weeks after acute SCI
- Resorptive hypercalciuria
- Hypercalcemia could be present, particularly in young individuals.
- Significant difference in bone mineral content (BMC) in the upper limbs between quadriplegics and paraplegics—higher in paraplegics

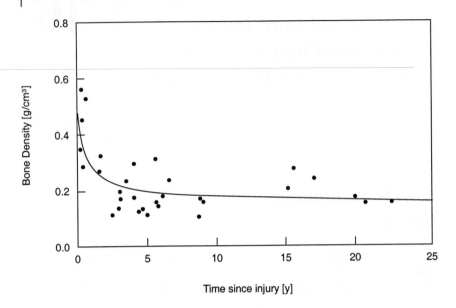

Figure 1: Trabecular bone density at the distal end of the fibia in a group of spinal-cord injured (SCI) patients, plotted against the time since injury. The data show a considerable amount of variability, as is to be expected in these patients. A regression line based on an exponential function, however, can provide the pattern of bone loss to be expected in pafients with spinal cord injury. (Adapted from Hangartner TN. Osteoporosis Due to Disuse. In: *Physical Medicine and Rehabilitation Clinics of North America.* Matkovic V. (Ed.). Philadelphia: Saunders, 1995;579–593.

- No loss of BMD in lumbar spine in paraplegics
- Increased incidence of long bone fractures with trivial trauma
- Fractures can occur during normal events in rehabilitation, e.g., transfer activity and range of motion.

Diagnosis

- Plain x-ray, dual energy x-ray absorptiometry (DXA), peripheral quantitative computerized tomography (pQCT).

Treatment

- Generally not satisfactory
- Calcitonin; bisphosphonates
- Functional electrical stimulation

Renal Calculi

- Overall incidence of urinary tract stones is 17.7%; renal stones 14.8%
- Type of stones: magnesium ammonium phosphate (struvite), calcium phosphate, calcium oxalate

- Contributing factors: hypercalcemia, vesicoureteral reflex, urinary tract infection with urea splitting bacteria; foley or suprapubic catheters.
- Calcium and magnesium ammonium phosphates precipitate in the alkaline medium. A nidus is formed on which more crystals deposit, eventually forming staghorn calculi.

Prevention

- Intermittent catheterization, appropriate diuresis, effective treatment of infections

Treatment

- Renal and bladder calculi usually found in the SCI population fragment easily.
- Lithotripsy is the treatment of choice for partial staghorn calculi.
- For complete staghorn calculi, percutaneous nephrolithotomy followed by lithotripsy is the treatment of choice.

Heterotopic Ossification (HO)

- Incidence is 10–53%.
- Etiology unclear, but central and local mechanisms may be involved. Hormonal, genetic, and metabolic causes are postulated.
- Microtrauma around the affected joint is implicated, aggressive rehabilitation including range of motion is thought to be contributory.
- Pressure sores, immobilization, infection and vasomotor disturbances are associated with HO.

Diagnosis

- Triple phase bone scan positive in early stage; however, may not be positive in the first few days of the inflammatory process.
  - Disadvantages of bone scan: uses ionizing radiation; expensive; not portable to bedside
- Ultrasound is positive in early stages of HO and is the least expensive method of detection. Usually it is positive at the time of first clinical symptoms. It has very characteristic appearance depending on the age and stage of mineralization of the lesion. Early findings include zone phenomena. With bone maturation, zone phenomena disappear and ultrasound beam is reflected in characteristic fashion.
- Increased serum alkaline phosphatase, as well as increased excretion of urinary prostaglandins (PGE_2).
- Plain x-rays positive but only 4–6 weeks after first clinical symptoms of HO.

Treatment

- Various regimens including biphosphonates alone, nonsteroidal anti-inflammatory drugs (NSAIDS, indomethacin) alone, or biphosphonates in combination with NSAIDS (intravenous disodium etidronate 300 mg/day for 3 days, followed by oral dose of 20 mg/kg/day for 6 months). Newer biphosphonates should be considered as well.

- Warfarin may be useful in prophylaxis against HO.
- Radiation therapy is an effective modality.
- Surgical resection of HO can result in recrudescence. Prophylactic presurgical and postsurgical treatment is recommended. Disodium etidronate alone or in combination with NSAIDS is effective prophylaxis for surgery.

Hypercalcemia

- Occurs mostly in young SCI patients (growing skeleton with increased number of bone remodeling units). It is caused by the excessive bone resorption acutely during the disease (first 3–6 months).

Treatment

- Hydration, forced diuresis, calcitonin, biphosphonates.

Traumatic Brain Injury

- The most important complication related to bone tissue in persons who have sustained traumatic brain injury (TBI), is heterotopic bone formation. Most likely explanation: a certain growth factor released by neurotrauma triggers osteogenic potential of mesenchymal stem cell (MSC) locally in the soft tissue.
- Reported incidence of HO in TBI is from 11–76%.
- Coma or vegetative state lasting one month or more is associated with significantly increased risk of HO. Spasticity is a contributory factor.
- Onset of HO is usually 4 to 12 weeks after TBI.
- Treatment is same as for HO occurring in SCI detailed above.

References

1. Banovac K, Gonzalez F, Wade N, Bowker JJ. Intravenous disodium etidronate therapy in spinal cord injury patients with heterotopic ossification. *Paraplegia* 1993;31(10):660–6.

2. Bienng-Sorensen F, Bohr HH, Schaadt OP. Longitudinal study of bone mineral content in the lumbar spine, the forearm, and the lower extremities after spinal cord injury. *Eur J Clin Invest* 1990;20(3):330–5

3. Cassar-Pulchino VN, McClelland M, Badwan DA, McCall IW, Pringle RG, el Masry W. Sonographic diagnosis of heterotopic bone formation in spinal injury patients. *Paraplegia* 1993;3 1(1):40–50.

4. Go BK, DeVivo MJ, Richards S. The Epidemiology of Spinal Cord Injury. In: Stover SL, DeLisa JA, Whiteneck GG, (eds). *Spinal Cord Injury. Clinical Outcomes from the Model Systems.* Gaithersburg: Aspen, 1995:21–55.

5. Hall MK, Hackler RH, Zampieri TA, Zampieri JB. Renal calculi in spinal cord injured patient: association with reflux, bladder stones, and foley catheter drainage. *Urology* 1989;34(3):126–8.

6. Schurch B, Capaul M, Vallotton MB, Rossier AB. Prostaglandin E2 measurements: Their value in the early diagnosis of heterotopic ossification in spinal cord injury patients. *Arch Phys Med Rehabil* 1997;78:687–91.

Reflex Sympathetic Dystrophy

Definition

- Reflex sympathetic dystrophy (RSD) is a syndrome characterized by diffuse limb pain, swelling, vasomotor and sudomotor phenomena, hyperalgesia, allodynia and trophic changes. The exact pathophysiology of RSD is still unclear. An inciting traumatic event is usually, but not always identifiable. Trauma may be major or very trivial. Fractures or ankle sprains frequently precede RSD. Several other events have been associated with RSD including stroke, myocardial infarction, cancer, surgery, and even the use of antituberculosis medications. Transient regional osteoporosis is a form of RSD.
- The International Association for the Study of Pain (IASP) issued a consensus statement redefining RSD in 1993. RSD is now grouped as a member of the complex regional pain syndromes (CRPS). It is designated CRPS type I. To avoid confusion, the term RSD is used here.
- The clinical features of causalgia are very similar to RSD.
- A major differentiating point between RSD (CRPS I) and causalgia (CRPS II) is that causalgia is usually associated with a partial nerve injury. In RSD, injury to a named nerve is not usually present.

Diagnosis

- The diagnosis is made based on clinical signs and symptoms (*dolor, tumor, calor, rubor, functio laesa*).
- There is spontaneous pain beyond the territory of a single peripheral nerve. The pain is disproportionate to the noxious event.
- Abnormal sudomotor and or vasomotor activity and swelling of skin and subcutaneous tissues usually follows. There is dysregulation of blood flow and sweating.
- Spontaneous pain, allodynia, hyperalgesia, hyperpathia are present.
- Trophic changes of skin, appendages of skin, subcutaneous tissue and bone atrophy develop at later stage.
- A single limb is affected initially, maximally so in the distal portion. Movement disorders including increased physiological tremor, spasm and dystonia occur.
- The number of symptoms and the extent to which each is expressed is quite variable.
- Plain x-ray shows patchy osteoporosis.

Diagnostic Procedures

- No single test is diagnostic of RSD, but a number of laboratory tests, in conjunction with clinical criteria mentioned above, help clinch the diagnosis.
  - Skin surface temperature measurement is helpful. Digital pad surfaces are used The normal and affected extremities are compared. Measurements are made symmetrically using infrared thermography. Environmental temperature should be well controlled and stable before measurements. Temperature difference >2° C is suggestive of unilateral sympathetic dysfunction.
  - Sympathetic blocks: Successful response to sympathetic blockade (pain relief) indicates that a component of, if not all of, the person's pain is mediated by the

sympathetic nervous system. This is defined as sympathetically maintained pain (SMP). A positive response to sympathetic blockade supports treatment directed to the sympathetic system. A negative response to sympathetic blockade indicates sympathetically independent pain (SIP). In SIP, treatment directed to the sympathetic nervous system is unlikely to be rewarding. The quantitative sudomotor axon reflex test (QSART) measures evoked sweat response. It measures resting cholinergic sympathetic tone and sudomotor activity stimulated by 10% acetylcholine per iontophoresis. A positive result for sympathetic overactivity shows increased sweat output and changes in latency and duration.

– Bone scan: Usually shows increased periarticular uptake.
– Quantitative bone mineral analysis by DXA shows decreased bone mineral content secondary to osteoporosis.
– X-rays may show bone demineralization similar to atrophy associated with immobilization or disuse. At first, there is a soft tissue swelling, and then diffuse periarticular osteopenia. Cortical bone resorption, subperiosteal, endosteal and intracortical. Articular erosions; metacarpophalangeal, metatarsophalangeal, proximal interphalangeal, and distal interphalangeal. X-ray findings proceed in stages.

Treatment

• No one method of treatment is guaranteed to succeed in treating RSD. Widely different pharmacological approaches may succeed in individual cases. Physical medicine and rehabilitation help. The wide range of successful treatments seems to imply different pathophysiological mechanisms for RSD.
• The mainstay of treatment is sympathetic blockade (usually with local anesthetic) a series of 1–6 blocks, one or more weeks apart, depending on the patient's response. For the upper limb, the stellate ganglion is the usual target. In the lower limb, the lumbar sympathetic chain is targeted.
  – Sympathetic blockade continues only if there is demonstrated response to the first block and subsequent blocks.
• Another approach is to employ pulse steroid therapy, e.g., with prednisone at high dose (100 mg orally/day), and decreasing by 10 mg each day till at zero. There is a good response to steroids especially in patients with the shoulder hand syndrome variety of RSD, treated early.
• Physical and occupational therapy are indispensable to increase functional use of the affected extremity. Maximal functional gain anticipated when the person afflicted with RSD is engaged in an active therapy program. Therapy should be employed immediately after pain relieving measures have been employed (sympathetic blocks, steroids etc.).
  – Stress loading of the affected limb
  – Range of motion of the limb
  – Transcutaneous neurostimulation and dorsal column stimulation could be applied as well.
• The most important consideration is adequate pain relief. If pain is not aggressively and effectively managed, there is little hope for restoring functional activity or reversing RSD.

Pharmacology

- Alpha-adrenergic blockers
- Gabapentin
- Mexiletine
- Biphosphonates
- Calcitonin
- Oral analgesics
- Intrathecal morphine

References

1. Baron R, Blumberg H, Janig W. Clinical Characteristics of Patients with Complex Regional Pain Syndrome in Germany with Special Emphasis on Vasomotor Function, In: Stanton-Hicks M, Janig W (eds) *Reflex Sympathetic Dystrophy: A Reappraisal*. Seattle: IASP Press, 1996;25–48.

2. Genant HK, Kozin F, Bekerman C, McCarty DJ, Sims J. The reflex sympathetic dystrophy syndrome. A comprehensive analysis using fine-detall radiography, photon absorptiometry, and bone and joint scintigraphy. *Radiology* 1975;117(1):2 1–32.

3. Low PA, Wilson PR, Sandroni P, Willner CL, Chelimsky TC. Clinical Characteristics of Patients with Reflex Sympathetic Dystrophy (Sympathetically Maintained Pain) in the USA. In: Stanton-Hicks M, Janig W, (eds). *Reflex Sympathetic Dystrophy: A Reappraisal*. Seattle:IASP Press, 1996;49–66.

17

Prevention of Bone Loss

Marjorie Luckey

Components of Prevention

- Maximize peak bone mass
  - Determined primarily by genetic factors
  - Can be influenced by diet, exercise, and lifestyle factors
- Prevent bone loss at every age

Maximize Peak Bone Mass in Children and Adolescents

- Calcium
  - Higher calcium intake increases bone mass during growth
  - Recommended intake
    - children, 800–1000 mg/day; adolescents, 1200 mg/day
  - Dairy products preferred because of accompanying protein
  - Use calcium supplements if intake is inadequate
- Exercise
  - Most effective in increasing bone mass during growth
  - Must continue through adolescence to have sustained effect
- Discourage excessive thinness
  - Direct correlation between body weight and bone mass
  - May lead to estrogen deficiency
- Stop smoking
  - Decreases circulating levels of estrogen
  - Toxic effect on osteoblasts
  - Contributes to low body weight
- Treat sex-hormone deficiency if it develops
  - Normal estrogen levels required for pubertal increase in bone density and attainment of adequate peak bone mass
  - Girls at risk for estrogen deficiency
    - excessively thin or with eating disorders
    - excessive exercise
    - glucocorticoid therapy
    - delayed menarche
    - genetic diseases (Turner's syndrome)/hypothalamic lesions

Prevention of Bone Loss

Men and Premenopausal Women

- Calcium
  - 1000 mg/day
  - Supplements if intake is inadequate
- Vitamin D
  - 200-400 IU/day
  - Supplement in winter or if sun exposure (w/o sunscreen) <15 minutes/day
- Exercise
  - Regular weight-bearing (walking, stair climbing, racket sports, skiing, etc.)
  - Muscle strengthening (i.e., exercise against resistance—swimming, weight training, rowing, etc.)
- Avoid smoking and excessive ETOH
- Consider bone densitometry if there are medical conditions or medications which cause rapid bone loss and osteoporosis

Postmenopausal Women

- Calcium
  - 1200–1500 mg/day
  - Supplements often required
    - calcium carbonate must be taken with food
    - calcium citrate produces less constipation and gas/absorbed with or without food/more expensive
- Vitamin D
  - 400 IU/day in healthy women
  - 800–1000 IU/day in housebound elderly or chronically ill adults
  - avoid intakes >1200 IU/day without regular monitoring
- Exercise (weight-bearing and muscle strengthening)
- Antiresorptive agents for women with
  - Low bone density
  - Major risk factors for osteoporosis

Indications for Bone Densitometry

Men and Premenopausal Women

- Medical conditions or medications associated with osteoporosis
- Results will influence Rx

Perimenopausal and Postmenopausal Women

- Family history of osteoporosis or fractures
- Low trauma fracture as adult
- Early menopause or history of prolonged oligo-amenorrhea
- 5–10 years postmenopause, not on HRT
- Low body weight (<125 lbs)

- Smoking
- Prolonged calcium-deficient diet
- Medical conditions or use of medications associated with osteoporosis

FDA Approved Agents

Prevention

- Estrogen replacement
- Alendronate, 5 mg/day
- Raloxifene, 60 mg/day

Treatment

- Estrogen replacement
- Alendronate, 10 mg/day
- Calcitonin, 200 IU/day IN; 100 IU/day SC

Estrogen Replacement

Effects on Bone

- Decreases bone resorption
- Prevents bone loss in both trabecular and cortical bone
- Decreases fracture incidence by 50% at all skeletal sites
- Increases bone density of the spine (5–6%) and hip (2–3%)
  - Greatest increases in women with recent or rapid bone loss
- Effective at all ages
- Most effective when combined with high calcium intake

Other Benefits

- Relieves menopausal symptoms
- May reduce cardiovascular mortality
- Improves lipid profile
  - Reduces total and LDL cholesterol
  - Increases HDL cholesterol
- Reduces risk of colon cancer
- Possible beneficial effect on memory

Available Preparations

- Oral, transdermal, implants, or vaginal preparations can be used
- Estrogens approved for osteoporosis prevention
  - Conjugated estrogen (Premarin, PremPro, PremPhase) 0.625 mg
  - Esterified estrogens (Estratab, Estratest) 0.3 and 0.625 mg
  - Estradiol patch(Estraderm) 0.05 mg
  - Estropipate (Ogen, Ortho-Est) 0.625
  - Micronized estradiol (Estrace) 0.5 mg

- Lower doses, in combination with calcium, may be adequate in some women
  - Follow-up with bone densitometry if lower doses are used
- Higher doses may be required in some women

Choosing an Estrogen Preparation

- Side effects of preparations vary in individuals
  - Try a different estrogen if side effects occur
- Oral estrogen is preferred route if well tolerated
  - Greater effect on lipid profile than transdermal estrogen
  - Most data on cardiovascular disease protection with oral ERT
- Transdermal estrogen preferred if:
  - High triglycerides
  - Liver disease
  - Gallbladder disorder
  - Malabsorption

Progestins

- Add to estrogen replacement to prevent endometrial hyperplasia
  - Unnecessary in women who have had a hysterectomy
- May be prescribed with estrogen as continuous (daily) or cyclic (10–14 days/month) regimen
  - May reduce estrogen's beneficial effects on lipids
  - Occasionally associated with premenstrual symptoms
- Available Progestins
  - Micronized progesterone
    - (100 mg bid for 12 days/month)
    - vaginal gel (6 applications over 12 days)
    - least adverse effect on lipids
    - may cause drowsiness
  - Medroxyprogesterone acetate
    - 5–10 mg for 12–14 days/month or 2.5–5 mg daily
  - Norethindrone acetate
    - 5 mg for 12–14 days/month or 1 mg daily

Side Effects

- Breast stimulation
  - Mastodynia and/or increased breast size
  - Possible small increase in risk of breast cancer with long term use
- Endometrial stimulation
  - Increased risk of endometrial hyperplasia and cancer if estrogen is used alone
    - risk not increased if adequate dose of progestin is added
  - Return of menses with cyclic progestin
  - Breakthrough bleeding frequent in first 6 months of daily combined estrogen and progestin
- Slight increase in risk of venous thrombotic events
- Increase in serum triglycerides

Contraindications

- Undiagnosed vaginal bleeding
- Estrogen dependent malignancy
- Acute, active liver disease
- Venous thrombosis or embolism on estrogen
- Severe hypertriglyceridemia

Raloxifene Hydrochloride (Evista)

- Selective Estrogen Receptor Modulator (SERM)
  - Estrogen-like effects on bone and lipids
  - No stimulation of endometrium or breast
  - No relief of menopausal symptoms
- FDA approved for osteoporosis prevention only
  - Not approved for treatment of established osteoporosis
- Recommended dose is 60 mg/day
  - No dietary restrictions
  - Concomitant progestin not required
  - High calcium intake recommended for maximum benefit on bone

Skeletal Effects

- Reduces bone resorption
- Prevents postmenopausal bone loss in spine and hip
  - Slight increase in density of hip (1.5%) and spine (1.5%)
    - increase in bone density is less than with ERT
  - Inconsistent effect on forearm (cortical) bone density
- Reduces risk of spine fracture by ~50%
  - No data available on hip fracture reduction

Breast

- No increase in breast tenderness
- Decreased breast cancer in clinical trials to date
  - Acts as estrogen antagonist on breast cancer cells in vitro
  - No data available regarding safety in women with past breast cancer

Genitourinary System

- No endometrial stimulation
  - No increase in vaginal bleeding
  - No endometrial hyperplasia
- No improvement in vaginal lubrication or atrophy

Lipids
- Decreases total and LDL cholesterol
- No increase in triglycerides
- No increase in HDL cholesterol

Vasomotor Symptoms
- Can increase hot flashes

Cardiovascular
- Increased incidence of venous thrombotic events (DVT and PE) comparable to estrogen
- No data on incidence of atherosclerosis or coronary artery disease
- Did not protect against coronary artery plaque formation in one monkey model

Other Effects
- Increased incidence of leg cramps
- No cognitive or psychomotor effects identified to date

Alendronate (Fosamax)

Third Generation Bisphosphonate
- Binds to hydroxyapatite on bone surfaces
- Decreases the number and activity of osteoclasts
- Inhibits bone resorption
- Results in histologically normal bone
- Long skeletal retention time

5 Mg Daily Prevents Bone Loss
- Increases bone density in spine (3–4%) and hip (1–2%)
  - 86% of subjects had some increase in bone density
- Reduces bone loss in forearm by 50%
- FDA approved for prevention of osteoporosis

10 Mg Daily Indicated for Treatment of Established Osteoporosis
- Increases bone density in spine (7–10%) and hip (5–7%)
- Reduces fractures by 50%

Important Instructions to Patients
- Take tablet upon rising with 6–8 oz plain water
- **Do not lie down** until after first meal
- Wait at least 30 minutes before taking food, beverage, or other medications

Cautions and Side Effects

- Poorly absorbed from GI tract
  - Must be taken on empty stomach
  - No food, drink, or medication for at least 30 minutes
- Musculoskeletal discomfort
  - No associated biochemical, local or systemic abnormalities
  - Frequently resolves despite continuing alendronate
- Potential irritant effect on esophagus and stomach
  - Some reports of esophogeal and gastric erosions and ulceration
    - increased incidence if dosing instructions not followed
    - increased risk with preexisting esophageal abnormalities
    - high risk of serious complications if drug continued after symptoms develop

Contraindications to Alendronate

- Active upper GI disease
- Structural abnormalities of esophagus
  - Strictures
  - Variceas or sclerotherapy
  - Acholasia
- Low serum calcium
  - Suggests other causes of bone disease
  - Correct before beginning antiresorptive therapy
- Renal insufficiency (creatinine clearance <30ml/min)
  - Excretion of drug is primarily renal
  - Drug not yet studied in renal failure

18

Prevention of Fractures in Patients with Low Bone Mass

Susan L. Greenspan

General Information
- One-third of people >65 year fall annually
- 90% of hip fractures occur after a fall
- Less than 5% of falls result in hip fractures

Controlled Clinical Trials
- Calcium and Vitamin D
  - Calcium 1200 mg/day and vitamin D 800 IU/day in nursing home or frail elderly for 1.5 years resulted in 43% reduction in hip fracture (Chapuy, 1992)
- External Hip Protector
  - Hip pads for one year in nursing home residents resulted in a 56% reduction in hip fractures (Lauritzens, 1993)
- Alendronate
  - Alendronate 10 mg/day for 3 years in postmenopausal women resulted in a 50% reduction in hip fractures (Black, 1993)

Medications Associated with Falls and Fractures
- Long-acting hypnotics
- Tricyclic antidepressants
- Antipsychotics
- Medications causing postural hypotension, confusion, dizziness, stiffness, and peripheral edema

Medical Factors Contributing to Falls and Fractures
- Postural hypotension
- Sway
- Sensory, motor, and vestibular malfunction
- Poor balance
- Unsteady gait/lower limb dysfunction
- Slow reaction time
- Visual impairment
- Poor hearing
- Cognitive impairment
- Impaired thermogenesis

The Bone and Mineral Manual
Copyright ©1999 by Academic Press
All rights of reproduction in any form reserved.

Biomechanical Risk Factors for Hip Fracture Independent of Low Bone Mass

- A sideways fall with impact on hip or side of leg
- Thin body habitus with less trochanteric soft tissue
- Poor protective responses to prevent fall

Multifactorial Intervention to Reduce Risk of Falls Among Community-Dwelling Elderly

- Controlled multifactorial intervention (Tinetti, 1994) reduced falls 30% over one year in 301 elderly over 70 years
- The intervention included 3 major domains
  1. Medication adjustments (eliminate sedatives and hypnotics; eliminate or adjust medications causing postural hypotension)
  2. Environmental evaluation (grab bars, raised toilet seats, handrails, safer furniture, remove hazards)
  3. Exercise and physical therapy (gait training, balance and strengthening exercises, appropriate assistive devices)

General Preventive Measures to Maintain Skeletal Integrity

- Encourage appropriate calcium intake (1000–1500 mg/day in divided doses)
- Encourage appropriate vitamin D intake (400 IU/day; 800 IU/day for elderly)
- Encourage weight-bearing exercise (walking 30 minutes 3 times per week) or high-intensity strength training (resistance training)
- Encourage therapy when appropriate to improve hip bone mineral density or prevent bone loss (hormone replacement therapy, alendronate, raloxifene)

General Preventive Measures to Prevent Falls and Fractures

Medical Assessment

- Maximize vision, hearing, lower extremity strength
- Correct underlying medical problems (i.e., heart failure, peripheral edema, Parkinson's disease, vitamin B_{12} deficiency, malnutrition, foot problems, hypotension)
- Review medications (eliminate long-acting sedatives, hypnotics, or those that cause confusion, dizziness, postural hypotension, stiffness, and peripheral edema)

Physical Therapy/Exercise Assessment

- Balance and strengthening exercises
- Gait assessment
- Appropriate assistive devices (cane, walker)
- Exercise (walking 30 minutes 3 times per week, high-intensity strength training or resistance training)

Occupational Therapy Assessment

- Environmental safety
- Home assessment (safe house)

Home Safety Measures to Prevent Falls

General

- Good lighting
- Clutter-free environment
- Avoid scatter rugs
- Remove loose wires and cords
- No slippery floors
- Supportive low-heeled shoes

Bathroom

- Grab bars in bathtub/shower
- No-skid mats

Bedroom

- Good lighting by bed
- Phone by bed

Stairs

- Well-lit
- Handrails both sides

References

1. Black DM, Cummings SR, Karpf DB, et al. for the Fracture Intervention Trial Research Group. Randomised trial of effect of alendronate on risk of fracture in women with existing vertebral fractures. *Lancet* 1996;348:1535–1541.

2. Chapuy MC, Arlot ME, Duboeuf F, et al. Vitamin D_3 and calcium to prevent hip fractures in elderly women. *N Engl J Med* 1992;327:1637–1642.

3. Cummings SR, Nevitt MC, Browner WS, et al. for the Study of Osteoporotic Fractures Research Group. Risk factors for hip fracture in white women. *N Engl J Med* 1995;332: 767–773.

4. Greenspan SL, Myers ER, Maitland LA, Resnick NM, Hayes WC. Fall severity and bone mineral density as risk factors for hip fracture in ambulatory elderly. *JAMA* 1994;271: 128–133.

5. Grisso JA, Kelsey JL, Strom BL, et al. and the Northeast Hip Fracture Study Group. Risk factors for falls as a cause of hip fracture in women. *N Engl J Med* 1991;324:1326–1331.

6. Lauritzen JB, Petersen MM, Lund B. Effect of external hip protectors on hip fractures. *Lancet* 1993;341:11–13.

7. Melton III LJ, Riggs BL. Risk factors for injury after a fall. *Clin Geriatr Med* 1985; 1:525–539.

8. Ray WA, Griffin MR, Schaffner W, Baugh DK, Melton III LJ. Psychotropic drug use and the risk of hip fracture. *N Engl J Med* 1987;316:363–369.

9. Resnick NM, Greenspan SL. Senile osteoporosis reconsidered. *JAMA* 1989;261:1025–1029.

10. Tinetti ME, Baker DI, McAvay G, et al. A multifactorial intervention to reduce the risk of falling among elderly people living in the community. *N Engl J Med* 1994;331:821–827.

Evaluation

Robert Marcus
Michael Kleerekoper
Ethel S. Siris

19

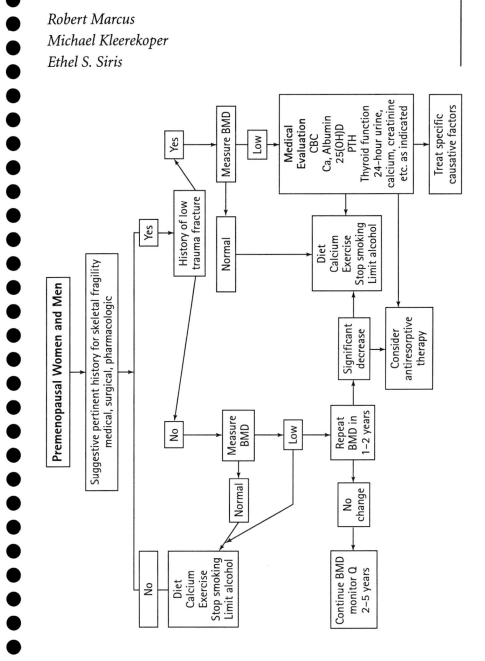

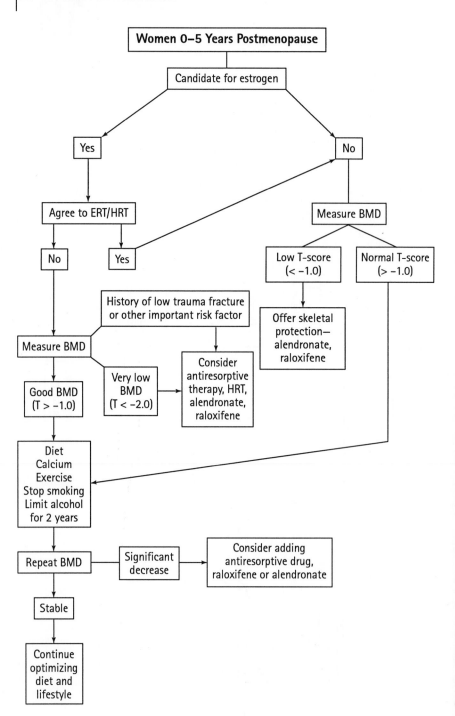

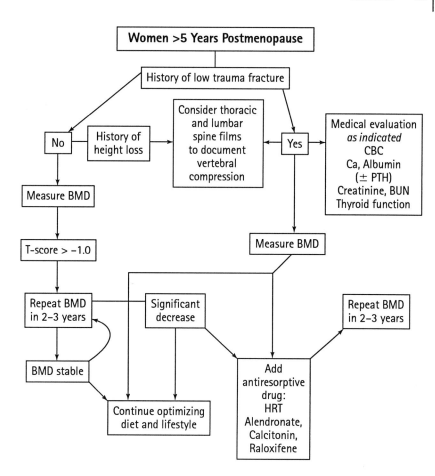

20

Osteoporosis in Men

Eric Orwoll

Clinical Impact *(Data reflect North American and Northern European experience)*

- Approximately 20% of the total health care costs of osteoporosis can be attributed to fractures in men.
- The lifetime risk of sustaining a nontraumatic fracture in a 60-year-old man is approximately 25%.
- The age-adjusted male/female incidence ratio for hip fracture is about 1:2.
- Because more women live to older age, ~80% of hip fractures are in women.

Clinical Characteristics

- Most men who experience osteoporotic fractures are elderly. The average age of hip fracture is about 80. There is a rapid increase in the incidence of vertebral and hip fractures beginning at about age 70.
- Two-thirds of men who present with osteoporotic fractures will have identifiable causes of metabolic bone disease. One-third are "idiopathic."
- Common causes of osteoporosis in men are glucocorticoid excess, alcohol excess, and hypogonadism.
- Other contributing causes include renal stone disease, malabsorption, smoking, anticonvulsants, etc.

Predictors of Fracture Risk

- Few longitudinal studies that definitively identify predictors of fracture in men.
- Strong candidates include:
  - Low bone mineral density
  - Previous fractures (vertebral or appendicular)
  - Increased likelihood of falling
  - Family history of fracture
  - Low body weight and weight loss
- These risk factors can be used in clinical situations to identify patients who need more aggressive diagnostic, preventive, and therapeutic attention.

The Bone and Mineral Manual
Copyright ©1999 by Academic Press

Determinants of Bone Mass

- Most studies currently available are cross-sectional evaluations of relatively small populations.
- Correlates of higher bone mass include:
  - Weight
  - Thiazide use
  - Strength/physical activity
- Lower bone mass is related to:
  - Aging
  - Inactivity
  - Smoking
  - Heavy alcohol intake
  - Glucocorticoids
  - Low sex steroid levels
  - Hypercalciuria
  - Low calcium intake
  - Vitamin D insufficiency
  - Anticonvulsants

Hypogonadism

- Low sex steroid levels are associated with reduced bone mass. This may be especially true when hypogonadism is present during pubertal (peak) bone mass development.
- In its early stages, loss of gonadal function in men results in a high turnover form of bone loss similar to that seen in the early postmenopausal period.
- Common causes of low testosterone levels include:
  - Testicular disease
  - Pituitary insufficiency
  - Alcohol abuse
  - Glucocorticoid therapy
  - Androgen ablation as treatment for prostate cancer
  - Aging

Androgen Therapy

- Testosterone replacement therapy can result in reduced bone turnover and some gain in bone mass.
- Androgen therapy can also increase lean body mass and strength.
- In some illnesses associated with low testosterone levels (e.g., glucocorticoid excess), androgen replacement may have positive effects on bone.
- Adverse effects associated with androgen therapy may include prostate disease, erythrocytosis, and reduced HDL levels.

Evaluation

- A comprehensive history and physical should be designed to detect risk factors for bone loss and falling
- Routine laboratory evalution should include:
  - Serum calcium, phosphorus, albumin, creatinine, liver functions, alkaline phosphatase; CBC; serum protein electrophoresis (in older men)
  - Serum 25 (OH) vitamin D level
  - 24-hour urine calcium, creatinine
  - Serum free testosterone level

When to Measure BMD

- History of fracture
- Radiographic osteopenia or vertebral deformity
- Risk factors for bone loss or fracture

Routine Prevention/Therapy

- Optimize vitamin D (400–800 IU/day) and dietary calcium (1200 mg/day) intake.
- Optimize safe physical activity, preferably weight-bearing.
- Consider testosterone replacement for men with free testosterone levels below the normal range.
- Avoid risk factors for bone loss (smoking, excessive alcohol intake, inactivity, etc.).

Pharmacological Therapy

- There are no clinical trials to guide the use of available therapies (calcitonin, bisphosphonates).
- By extrapolation from experience in women, calcitonin and bisphosphonates may be effective in men.
- Consider pharmacological therapy in men with osteoporosis (BMD T score < –2.5) and in men with low bone mass (T score –1 to 2.5) plus risk factors for further bone loss.

21

Steroid-Induced Osteoporosis

Barbara P. Lukert

Glucocorticoid-Induced Osteoporosis

- Occurs in 30-50% of patients receiving long-term glucocorticoid therapy
- Trabecular bone lost more rapidly than cortical bone
- Loss is rapid, in some cases 20% in one year
- Bone loss may be greatest during first 6–12 months.

Effects of Glucocorticoids on Calcium Homeostasis and Bone Metabolism

- Inhibit GI absorption of calcium and cause hypercalciuria
- Induce secondary hyperparathyroidism
- Lower gonadal hormone levels
- Inhibit bone formation
- Cause aseptic necrosis

Interactions between Glucocorticoids and Other Factors

- Increase sensitivity of osteoblasts to PTH and $1,25(OH)_2D$
- Inhibit prostaglandin E production
- Decrease local (bone) production of IGF-1
- Alter IGF binding proteins
- Inhibit biologic effect of IGF-1
- Increase production of collagenase

Theories of Etiology of Aseptic Necrosis

- Vascular (fat emboli)
- Mechanical (accumulation of trabecular microcracks)
- Increased intraosseous pressure due to fat accumulation impinging on vascular bed

The Bone and Mineral Manual
Copyright ©1999 by Academic Press
All rights of reproduction in any form reserved.

Effects on Muscle

- Not dose dependent
- Creatinuria in presence of normal serum muscle enzymes
- Selective atrophy of type II fibers
- Loss of muscle strength
- Myalgia

Assessment of Patient Receiving Glucocorticoids

- Assess nutritional status, muscle strength, and mobility
- Bone mineral analysis of spine and hip
- X-rays of thoracic and lumbar spine
- 24-hour urine calcium, creatinine, and sodium
- Serum 25 (OH) vitamin D

Management

General Considerations

- Use lowest effective dose of glucocorticoid
- Use glucocorticoid with short half life
- Use topical steroids when possible
- Maintain highest possible level of physical activity

Prevent Secondary Hyperparathyroidism

- Control hypercalciuria and improve calcium absorption
  - Restrict sodium to 3 g/day
  - If still hypercalciuric, add thiazide and potassium-sparing diuretic.
- Assure calcium intake of 1500 mg/day
- Maintain serum 25 (OH) vitamin D at upper range of normal
  - Vitamin D supplement of 800 IU/day
  - May need higher dose if there are signs of malabsorption

Treat Hypogonadism

- **Postmenopausal women:** Estrogen/progesterone replacement if there are no contraindications
- **Premenopausal women:** If there are changes in menstrual periods, measure serum estradiol levels and cycle with estrogen/progesterone if levels are low.
- **Men:** Measure serum testosterone. If low, replace if there are no contraindications.

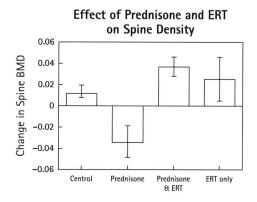

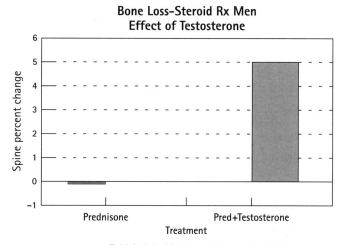

Reid, Arch Int Med, June 1996, reprinted with permission

Antiresorptive Drug Use

- Monitor bone density every 6 months for first 2 years
- If continuing to lose bone in spite of controlling calcium balance and treating hypogonadism, consider the following:
  - Bisphosphonates
    - Etidronate 400 mg for 2 weeks out of every 3 months has been shown to prevent bone loss.
    - Alendronate 10 mg daily prevents bone loss.
    - Nasal calcitonin 200 units/day probably prevents loss.

References

1. Adams JS, Wahl TO, Lukert BP. Effects of hydrochlorothiazide and dietary sodium restriction on calcium metabolism in corticosteroid treated patients. *Metabolism* 1981;30:217–221.

2. Crilly RG, Cawood M, Marshall DH, Nordin BE. Hormonal status in normal, osteoporotic and corticosteroid-treated postmenopausal women. *J R Soc Med* 1978;71:733–736.

3. Horber FF, Haymond MW. Human growth hormone prevents the protein catabolic side effects of prednisone in humans. *J Clin Invest* 1990;86:265–272.

4. Ip M, Lam K, Yam L, Kung A, Ng M. Decreased bone mineral density in premenopausal asthma patients on long-term inhaled steroids. *Chest* 1994;105:1722–1727.

5. Luengo M, Picado C, Del Rio L, Guanabens N, Monsterrat JM, Setoain J. Treatment of steroid-induced osteopenia with calcitonin in corticosteroid-dependent asthma: a one-year follow-up study. *Am Rev Respir Dis* 1990;142:104–107.

6. Lukert BP, Raisz LG. Glucocorticoid-induced osteoporosis: pathogenesis and management. *Ann Intern Med* 1990;112:352–364.

7. Lukert BP, Johnson BE, Robinson RG. Estrogen and progesterone replacement therapy reduces glucocorticoid-induced bone loss. *J Bone Miner Res* 1992;7(9):1063–1069.

8. Packe G, Douglas J, McDonald A, Robins S, Reid D. Bone density in asthmatic patients taking high dose inhaled beclomethasone dipropionate and intermittent systemic corticosteroids. *Thorax* 1992;47:414–417.

9. Puolijoki H, Liippo K, Herrala J, Salmi J, Tala E. Inhaled beclomethasone decreases serum osteocalcin in postmenopausal asthmatic women. *Bone* 1992;13:285–288.

10. Reid IR, Frances JT, Pybus J, Ibbertson HK. Low plasma testosterone levels in glucocorticoid-treated male asthmatics. *Brit Med J* 1985;291:574.

11. Reid I. Effect of testosterone on bone loss in steroid-treated men. *Arch Intern Med* June, 1996.

12. Rizzato G, Tosi G, Schiraldi G, Montemurro L, Zanni D, Sisti S. Bone protection with salmon calcitonin (sCT) in the long-term steroid therapy of chronic sarcoidosis. *Sarcoidosis* 1988;5:99–103.

13. Schwartzman MS, Franck WA. Vitamin D toxicity complicating the treatment of senile, postmenopausal, and glucocorticoid-induced osteoporosis. Four case reports and a critical commentary on the use of vitamin D in these disorders. *Am J Med* 1987;82:224–230.

14. Struys A, Anneke A, Mulder H. Cyclical etidronate reverses bone loss of the spine and proximal femur in patients with established corticosteroid-induced osteoporosis. *Am J Med* September, 1995.

22

Organ Transplantation

Elizabeth Shane

Epidemiology

- Approximately 132,000 solid organ transplants were performed in the United States alone between 1988 and 1995.
- Kidney transplants were most common (~62%) followed by liver, heart, pancreas, lung, and heart/lung.
- Five-year survival rates range from 97% for kidney to approximately 50% for heart/lung.
- Available data indicate that approximately 50% of organ transplant recipients have osteoporosis as defined by bone densitometry or fractures.
- Vertebral fracture prevalence ranges from 10–50%.

Risk Factors for Bone Loss Before Transplantation

- Kidney—intestinal calcium malabsorption, therapy with loop diuretics and/or glucocorticoids, secondary hyperparathyroidism, aplastic bone disease, chronic metabolic acidosis, hypogonadism
- Liver—alcoholism, primary biliary cirrhosis, hypogonadism, abnormal hepatic vitamin D metabolism
- Heart and Heart/Lung—vitamin D deficiency, secondary hyperparathyroidism, physical inactivity, therapy with loop diuretics, tobacco, alcoholism
- Lung—glucocorticoid therapy, tobacco, cystic fibrosis, physical inactivity, hypogonadism
- Pancreas—insulin-dependent diabetes mellitus

Risk Factors for Bone Loss After Transplantation

Glucocorticoids

- Generally prescribed in high doses immediately after transplantation (100 mg daily of prednisone or its equivalent) with gradual taper to 5–10 mg daily by 6 months.
- High doses with slightly more rapid taper is also the most common therapy for rejection.

- Recent trend toward somewhat lower doses and more rapid taper of glucocorticoids and attempts to withdraw patients by 6–12 months.
- Sufficient exposure in the first 6 months to cause bone loss even in programs that use lower doses of glucocorticoids.

Cyclosporines and Tacolimus (FK 506) Animal Studies

- Relatively brief administration of both cyclosporine A and (FK 506) associated with profound bone loss in animal studies.
- Bone resorption and formation both increased with resorption obviously exceeding formation.
- Skeletal effects likely mediated by increased expression of interleukin-1.
- Serum $1,25(OH)_2D$ and osteocalcin concentrations increased.
- Bone loss prevented by drugs that inhibit bone resorption (estrogen, calcitonin, alendronate, raloxifene).

Natural History of Bone Loss

- Bone loss at lumbar spine and femoral neck ranges from 3–20% during the first year after kidney, liver, and heart transplantation. Radial site generally not affected during the first year.
- Few prospective data in heart/lung, lung, or pancreas recipients
- Bone loss slows or stops in most, but not all, patients after the first year.
- Considerable variability in rates of bone loss among individuals

Natural History of Fracture

- Most common sites of fracture are vertebrae and ribs.
- Hip and sacral fractures also reported.
- Fracture incidence range from 5–65%.
- Liver, heart, and lung recipients have higher fracture rates than kidney recipients.
- Peak fracture incidence very early after transplantation, then declines.
- In one study, 85% sustained their initial fracture within the first 6 months after cardiac transplantation.
- Postmenopausal women have higher risk of fracture.
- Even patients with normal pretransplant bone mass fracture.
- No baseline densitometric or biochemical parameter predicts fracture in the individual.

Biochemical Correlates of Bone Loss

- Transient decrease in serum osteocalcin and increase in bone resorption markers, during first six months after cardiac transplantation.
- In men, transient decline in serum testosterone during first 6 months after cardiac transplantation.
- Rates of bone loss after cardiac transplantation directly correlated with:
  - Greater suppression of osteocalcin and testosterone
  - Lower levels of 25-hydroxyvitamin D and 1,25-dihydroxyvitamin D
  - Higher levels of bone resorption markers
  - Greater exposure to glucocorticoids

Principles of Management

- Significant osteopenia and abnormal bone and mineral metabolism often antedates transplantation. Therefore, all patients should be evaluated for osteoporosis at time of acceptance to waiting list.
- Most rapid rates of bone loss and highest fracture incidence occur during the first 6–12 months. Therefore, efforts to prevent these complications should begin *before or immediately after* transplantation.
- Patients with normal pretransplant bone mineral density fracture after transplantation. Therefore, prophylaxis of bone loss and fracture should be instituted in all organ transplant recipients, regardless of pretransplant BMD.

Pretransplant Evaluation

- History and physical examination with particular attention to risk factors for osteoporosis
- Bone mineral density of spine and hip
- Thoracic and lumbar spine radiographs
- Essential biochemistries: serum calcium, phosphorus, alkaline phosphatase, intact parathyroid hormone, 25-hydroxyvitamin D, thyroid function tests
- Optional biochemistries: markers of bone turnover such as serum osteocalcin or bone specific alkaline phosphatase, urinary calcium, n-telopeptide or pyridnium crosslink excretion

Pretransplant Management

- Begin RDA for calcium and vitamin D.
- Encourage weight-bearing and strengthening exercises.
- Treat hypogonadism with estrogen or androgen replacement if no contraindications.
- Treat pretransplant osteoporosis with appropriate medication (hormone replacement, bisphosphonates, calcitonin).

Prevention

General Principles

- Rapid resumption of weight-bearing exercise; enrollment in organized rehabilitation program after transplantation
- Rapid reduction of glucocorticoid dose as permitted by clinical situation
- Encourage alternative methods of handling rejection that do not involve high dose glucocorticoids

Specific Approaches

- Place all patients on elemental calcium (1000–1500 mg daily in divided doses) and at least 400–800 IU of vitamin D.
- Consider prescribing antiresorptive drugs (bisphosphonates, calcitonin, estrogen) as soon as practical after surgery.
- Pharmacologic doses of vitamin D [25 α calcidiol, 1,25(OH)$_2$ vitamin D] have also been shown to reduce bone loss.
- Fluoride would be a last choice.

Cautionary Note

- Renal transplant recipients must be managed with caution. Hypercalciuria must be avoided to preserve graft function. Certain bisphosphonates might exacerbate persistent posttransplant hypophosphatemia and hyperparathyroidism.

References

1. Aris RM, Neuringer IP, Weiner MA, Egan TM, Ontjes D. Severe osteoporosis before and after lung transplantation. *Chest* 1996;109:1176–1183.

2. Epstein S. Post-transplantation bone disease: the role of immunosuppressive agents on the skeleton. *J Bone Miner Res* 1996;11:1–7.

3. Epstein S, Shane E .Transplantation osteoporosis. In: Marcus R, Feldman D, Kelsey J, eds. *Osteoporosis*. New York: Academic Press. 1996;947–957.

4. Henderson NK, Sambrook PN, Kelly PJ, et al. Bone mineral loss and recovery after cardiac transplantation. *Lancet* 1995;ii:905.

5. Julian BA, Laskow DA, Dubovsky J, Dubovsky EV, Curtis JJ, Quarles LD. Rapid loss of vertebral bone density after renal transplantation. *New Engl J Med* 1991;325:544–550.

6. Lukert BP. Glucocorticoid-induced osteoporosis. In: Marcus R, Feldman D, Kelsey J, eds. *Osteoporosis*. New York: Academic Press. 1996;801–820.

7. Meys E, Fontanges E, Fourcade N, et al. Bone loss after orthotopic liver transplantation. *Am J Med* 1994;97:445–450.

8. Rich GM, Mudge GH, Laffel GL, LeBoff MS. Cyclosporine A and prednisone-associated osteoporosis in heart transplant recipients. *J Heart Lung Transplant* 1992;11:950–958.

9. Sambrook PN, Kelly PJ, Keogh A, et al. Bone loss after cardiac transplantation: a prospective study. *J Heart Lung Transplant* 1994;13:116–121.

10. Shane E, Epstein E. Immunosuppressive therapy and the skeleton. *Trends Endocrinol Metab* 1994;4:169–175.

11. Shane E, Rivas M, Silverberg SJ, et al. Osteoporosis after cardiac transplantation. *Am J Med* 1993;94:257–264.

12. Shane E, Rivas M, McMahon DJ, et al. Bone loss and turnover after cardiac transplantation. *J Clin Endocrinol Metab* 1997;82:1497–1506.

13. Shane E, Rivas M, Staron RB, et al. Fracture after cardiac transplantation: a prospective longitudinal study. *J Clin Endocrinol Metab* 1996;81:1740–1746.

14. Shane E, Thys-Jacobs S, Papadopoulos A, et al. Antiresorptive therapy prevents bone loss after cardiac transplantation. *J Heart Lung Transplant* in press, 1998.

15. Valero MA, Loinaz C, Larrodera L, et al. Calcitonin and bisphosphonate treatment and bone loss after liver transplantation. *Calcif Tissue Int* 1995;57:15–19.

23

Pharmacologic Therapy

Nelson B. Watts

General Measures for Osteoporosis

- **Calcium:** Diet is usually inadequate. The typical postmenopausal woman not taking estrogen needs a supplement of 1000 mg daily.
- **Vitamin D:** To assure adequacy, recommend 400–800 IU daily (1 or 2 multivitamin tabs).
- **Exercise:** Weight-bearing is best. Recommend walking 30 min. daily, 3–5 days per week.

Optimal Calcium Intake

- Adolescents   1500 mg daily
- Premenopausal women   1000 mg daily
- Postmenopausal not on estrogen   1500 mg daily
  - The average woman 50 and older gets less than 600 mg calcium daily from dietary sources, and thus needs a calcium supplement of almost 1000 mg daily.

Foods High in Calcium

- Skim milk, 1 cup   302 mg
- Nonfat yogurt, 1 cup   452 mg
- Cheddar cheese, 1oz   204 mg
- Frozen yogurt, 1/2 cup   154 mg
- Turnip greens, 1/2 cup   246 mg
- Sardines with bones, 2oz   217 mg
- Broccoli, 1/2 cup   89 mg

The Bone and Mineral Manual
Copyright ©1999 by Academic Press
All rights of reproduction in any form reserved.

Calcium Supplements

Calcium Salt	Calcium Content in 500 mg tab	Percent Calcium	Monthly Cost*
Carbonate	200 mg	40%	$ 3.00
Citrate	105 mg	21%	$ 6.00
Lactate	65 mg	13%	$ 6.00
Gluconate	45 mg	9%	$10.00

*Approximate cost for 1000 mg/day for 30 days, from *Consumer Reports*, August 1995; 510–513.

Postmenopausal Osteoporosis

Prevention of Bone Loss (also see Chapter 17)
• Estrogen
• Raloxifene
• Alendronate

Treatment of Osteoporosis
• Estrogen
• Calcitonin
• Alendronate

Estrogen for Osteoporosis

• Long-term ERT increases bone density and reduces the risk of osteoporotic fractures.

Additional Benefits of Estrogen
• Relieves symptoms of estrogen deficiency
• Reduces the risk of myocardial infarction

Other Important Considerations
• Migraine headaches
• Fibrocystic breast disease
• Uterine fibroids
• Endometriosis
• Venous thrombosis
• Continued menses
• Endometrial cancer
• Breast cancer

Underuse, Poor Compliance

- In the US, only about 15% of women who might benefit from estrogen are actually taking it.
- 30%–50% of prescriptions for estrogen are never filled.
- Only 20% of those who begin long-term HRT are still taking it 5 years later.

Problems

- Not recommended by physicians
- Patient does not understand need for long-term use
- Side effects (bleeding, breast tenderness, etc.)
- Unresolved concerns, HRT and breast cancer

Estrogen Prevents Bone Loss in Recently Oophorectomized Women

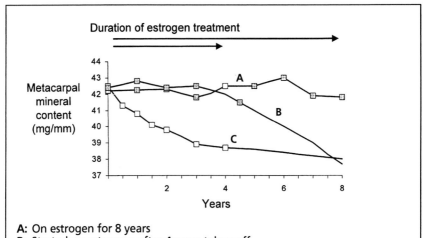

A: On estrogen for 8 years
B: Started on estrogen; after 4 years taken off.
C: Did not receive estrogen

Modified from Lindsay R et al, *Lancet* 1978;1:1325-1327

Effects of HRT on Bone Density—The Pepi Trial

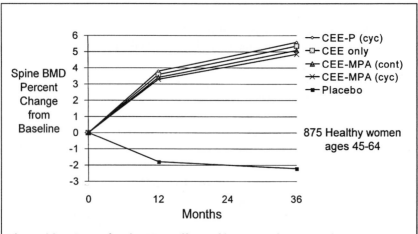

The Writing Group for the PEPI, *Effects of hormone therapy on bone mineral density. JAMA* 1996, 276(17):1389-96. Reprinted with permission.

Poor Long-Term Compliance with HRT

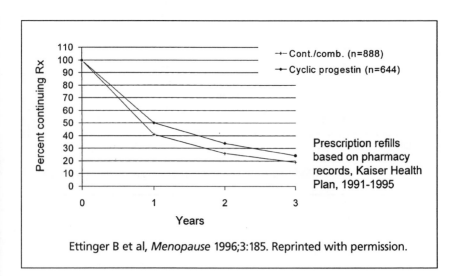

Ettinger B et al, *Menopause* 1996;3:185. Reprinted with permission.

Raloxifene for Osteoporosis

- The recommended dose is 60 mg daily.
- Prevents bone loss in recently menopausal women
- Positive effect on lipids (LDL, triglycerides)
- No uterine stimulatory effect
- Does not increase the risk of breast cancer
- Does not relieve hot flashes
- Small but significant incidence of DVT

Calcitonin for Osteoporosis

- Injectable salmon calcitonin available since 1984; not widely used because of high cost, discomfort, and side effects (nausea and/or flushing in ~20%)
- Nasal spray introduced; very well tolerated, recommended dose 200 IU daily
- Long-term safety is excellent.
- Analgesic effect makes calcitonin useful for patients with acute fracture or chronic pain.

Nasal Calcitonin—The PROOF Study

(Prevent Recurrence of Osteoporotic Fractures)

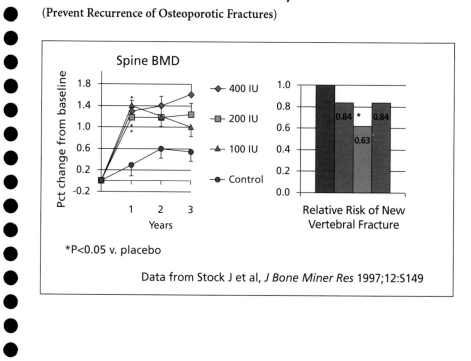

Data from Stock J et al, *J Bone Miner Res* 1997;12:S149

Nasal Calcitonin for Painful Vertebral Fracture

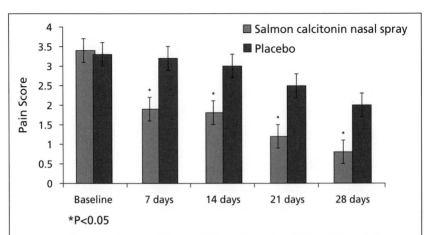

*P<0.05

Reprinted by permission of the publishers from Pun KK and Chan LW: Analgesia effect of intranasal salmon calcitonin in the treatment of osteoporotic vertebral fractures, *Clin Ther*, 11(2):205-09. ©1998 by Excerpta Medica Inc.

Bisphosphonates

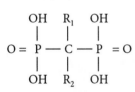

- Bone-seeking
- Effective orally or IV
- Poor absorption orally
- Not metabolized, excreted by the kidney
- Long skeletal retention
- Side chain determines potency

Generation	Side Chain	Relative Potency
• First	short alkyl or halide	1–10
– Etidronate		
– Clodronate		
• Second	amino terminal	100–1,000
– Tiludronate		
– Alendronate		
– Pamidronate		
• Third	cyclic	100,000–1,000,000
– Risedronate		
– Ibandronate		
– Zoledronate		

Alendronate Phase III Studies

- Two identical protocols conducted concurrently
  - (18 U.S. centers, 19 international)
- Three years, double-blind, placebo-controlled
- Subjects: 994 postmenopausal women with spine BMD T-score ≥2.5 SD
- Treatment Groups
  - Placebo
  - Alendronate 5 mg daily
  - Alendronate 10 mg daily
  - Alendronate 20 mg daily

Phase III Alendronate Study (U.S. Cohort)

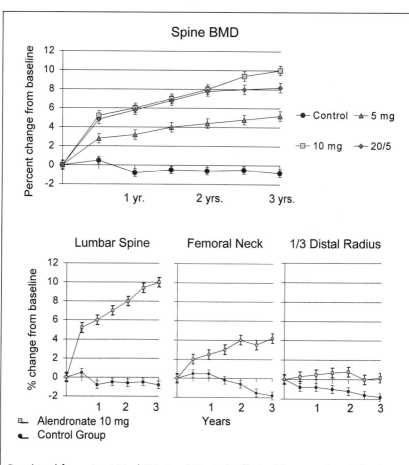

Reprinted from *Am J Med* 101, Tucci JR et al, Effect of 3 years of oral alendronate treatment in postmenopausal women with osteoporosis. Pp 488-501, 1996, with permission from Excerpta Medica Inc.

Fracture Intervention Trial (FIT)

- Age 55–80 with low femoral neck BMD placebo or alendronate 5mg/d for 2 years then 10 mg/day
- Arm 1: 2027 women with 1 or more vertebral fracture, followed for ~3 years (ended 2/96)
- Arm 2:4434 women without fracture, followed 4 to 4.5 years (complete 5/97)

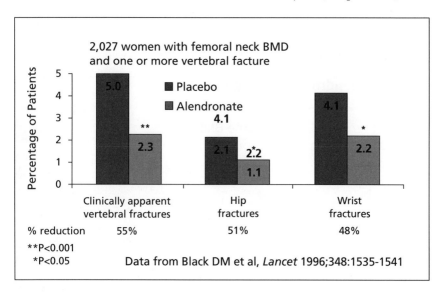

2,027 women with femoral neck BMD and one or more vertebral facture

Percentage of Patients

■ Placebo
■ Alendronate

	Clinically apparent vertebral fractures	Hip fractures	Wrist fractures
% reduction	55%	51%	48%

**P<0.001
*P<0.05

Data from Black DM et al, *Lancet* 1996;348:1535-1541

Alendronate Osteoporosis Prevention Studies

- 2357 patients
- Mean age 53 (range 40–59)
- Average 5 years postmenopause
- Exclusion criteria
  - Recent (in 1 year) major gastrointestinal disease
  - Regular use (>4 times/wk) of NSAIDs or ASA
  - Recent use of drug to inhibit gastric acid secretion

Early Postmenopausal Intervention Cohort (EPIC)

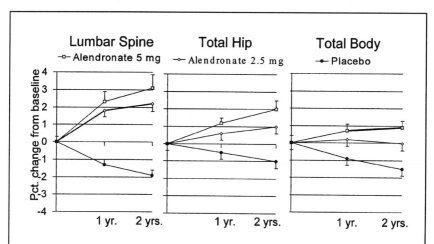

Data from Hosking D et al, Prevention of bone mass with alendronate in postmenopausal women under 60 years of age. *N Engl J Med* 1998, 338(8): 485-92.

Alendronate Dosing

- The recommended dose for treatment of postmenopausal osteoporosis is 10 mg daily.
- The dose for prevention of bone loss in recently menopausal women is 5 mg daily.
  - To be effective, it must be taken first thing in the morning, with water, but nothing else by mouth for at least 30 minutes.
  - For safety (to avoid esophageal irritation), the patient should remain upright (seated or standing) until she has eaten.

BMD Effects of Intermittent Cyclic Etidronate Plus Estrogen in 72 Postmenopausal Women

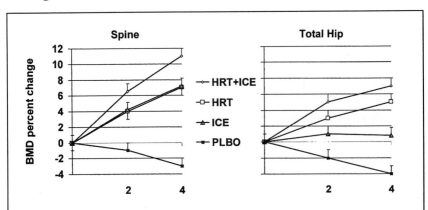

Reprinted from *Am J Med* 104. Wimalawansa S, A 4-year randomized controlled trial. Pp 219-226, 1998, with permission from Excerpta Medica Inc.

Miscellaneous Agents

- Androgens/anabolic steroids
- Ipriflavone
- Progestins
- Thiazide diuretics
- Tibolone
- Vitamin D metabolites/analogs
  - 25-hydroxyvitamin D
  - 1,25-dihydroxyvitamin D
  - 1α-hydroxyvitamin D

Potential New Agents

- New bisphosophonates
  - Risedronate
  - Ibandronate
  - Zoledronate
- New SERMs
- Parathyroid hormone
- Bone morphogenetic proteins
- Cytokines, cytokine inhibitors

24

Nonpharmacologic Therapy

Michael McClung

Objectives of Management

- Decrease incidence of fractures
  - Preserve or increase bone mass
  - Prevent injuries and falls
- Minimize symptoms
- Improve function and quality of life

Risk Factors for Fractures[1]

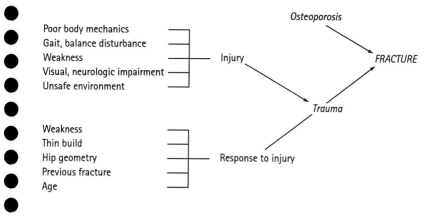

Treatment of Postmenopausal Osteoporosis

Exercise

- Weight-bearing exercise may optimize peak bone mass in young people.
- Immobilization in adults is associated with accelerated bone loss.
- Regular physical activity helps maintain bone mass but does not significantly increase BMD nor prevent bone loss.
- Most important role of exercise in older adults is to maintain muscle strength and function.

Calcium and Vitamin D Nutrition

- Adequate calcium and vitamin D intake
  - 1200–1500 mg total daily calcium intake for postmenopausal women
  - 1000 mg daily for men
  - Vitamin D 400-800 IU daily if over age 65
- Calcium and vitamin D therapy decrease hip fracture frequency in older women and nonvertebral fractures in older Americans.[2,3]
- Calcium decreases vertebral fracture incidence in women with previous fractures.[4]
- Protein administration improves bone density function after hip fracture.[5]

Fall and Injury Prevention[6]

- Maintain physical activity and strength
- Proper body mechanics; gait and balance training
- Ambulatory support when indicated
- Avoid sedative medications and excessive alcohol
- Minimize other contributing problems
- Safe home environment
- Hip protectors for frail elderly[7]

Symptom Control—Acute Vertebral Fracture

- Bed rest (for a few days)
- Gentle stretching exercises
- Heat, ice or physical therapy modalities if muscle spasm occurs
- Calcitonin nasal spray 200 units daily for 2 weeks if pain relief inadequate. If good response is apparent, continue for total of 6–8 weeks

Improving Chronic Back Pain and Function

- Generalized and targeted programs of exercise to stretch and strengthen extensor muscles of back[8,9]
- Appropriate analgesic or anti-inflammatory therapy
- Practical hints to cope with and to improve activities of daily living
- Reach extenders

Psychosocial Support[10]

- Review patient's living arrangements, family support and social network
- Listen to and validate concerns
- Educate about osteoporosis, nature of symptoms, expected outcomes
- Identify and discuss patient's objectives; set reasonable goals
- Group exercise class
- Osteoporosis support group

Summary

- There is more to treating patients with osteoporosis than just treating osteoporosis and low bone mass.
- Comprehensive patient management includes
  - Optimizing nutrition
  - Injury and fall prevention
  - Symptom control
  - Attending to functional and psychosocial limitations

References

1. Cummings SR, Nevitt MC, Browner WS, et al. Risk factors for hip fracture in white women. *N Engl J Med* 1995;332:767–773.

2. Chapuy MC, Arlot ME, Duboeuf F et al. Vitamin D$_3$ and calcium to prevent hip fractures in elderly women. *N Engl J Med* 1992;327:1637–1642.

3. Dawson-Hughes B, Harris D, Krall EA, Dallal GE. Effect of calcium and vitamin D supplementation on bone density in men and women 65 years of age or older. *N Engl J Med* 1997;337:670–676.

4. Recker RR, Hinders S, Davies KM, et al. Correcting calcium nutritional deficiency prevents spine fractures in elderly women. *J Bone Miner Res* 1996;11:1961–1966.

5. Schurch MA, Rizzoli R, Vidas L, et al. Protein supplements in elderly with a recent hip fracture increase serum IGF-l, decreases urinary deoxypyridinohne, and prevent proximal femur bone loss. *J Bone Miner Res* 1996;11:S139.

6. Tinnetti ME, Baker D, McAvay G, et al. Multifactorial intervention to reduce the risk of falling among elderly people living in the community. *N Engl J Med* 1994;331:821–827.

7. Lauritzen JB, Petersen MM, Lund B. Effect of external hip protectors on hip fractures. *Lancet* 1993;341:11–13.

8. Sinaki M. Musculo-skeletal rehabilitation. In: Riggs BI, Melton LJ, (eds), *Osteoporosis: Etiology, Diagnosis and Management.* 2nd Ed. Philadelphia: Lippincott-Raven Publishers 1995;435–473.

9. Harrison TE, Chou R, Dorman J, et al. Evaluation of a program for rehabilitation of osteoporotic patients: 4 year follow-up. *Osteoporosis Int* 1993;3:13–17.

10. Gold DT, Lyles KW, Bales CW, Drezner MK. Teaching patients coping behaviors: an essential part of successful management of osteoporosis. *J Bone Miner Res* 1989;4:799–801.

25

Paget's Disease

Ethel S. Siris

Epidemiology

- Both men and women affected, slight male predominance
- Affects 2–3% of people over age 55–60 in the United States.
- Clinical presentation usually occurs after age 45 to 50
- Most common in Caucasians of European ancestry
  - Less common in African-Americans
  - Rare in Asians

Pathophysiology

- Paget's disease is a localized disorder of bone remodeling affecting one or more bones or parts of bone.
- Osteoclasts at pagetic sites are increased in size and number.
- A slow virus (measles, respiratory syncitial, canine distemper?) and/or genetic factors (commonly runs in families) may cause the osteoclast abnormality.
- Increases in both osteoclastic bone resorption and subsequent new bone formation produces disordered bone architecture: lytic and sclerotic lesions, cortical thickening, trabecular coarsening, hypervascularity, and enlargement of bone.
- As a consequence of increased remodeling and architectural changes, Pagetic bone is prone to deformity and fracture.

Laboratory Tests

- Increased levels of bone resorption markers: urinary hydroxyproline, pyridinoline/deoxypyridinoline, n-telopeptide, c-telopeptide
- Increased levels of bone formation markers: serum alklaline phosphatase and bone specific alkaline phosphatase
- Serum calcium and phosphate normal
- Serum uric acid sometimes elevated
- Vitamin D metabolites normal, but PTH elevated in 15–20% of patients

The Bone and Mineral Manual
Copyright ©1999 by Academic Press
All rights of reproduction in any form reserved.

Radiology

- Bone scans: most sensitive for identifying affected sites, but not specific
- Radiographs: diagnostic of Paget's disease due to characteristic changes
  - Demonstrate degree of deformity, presence of dominant osteolytic lesions or fractures, status of adjacent joints
- CT or MR imaging: used primarily for assessment of neural compression syndromes, equivocal stress fractures, rare malignant complications

Clinical Presentation

- Many patients are asymptomatic when diagnosed.
- Signs and symptoms depend on sites of involvement, degree of deformity, and level of increased bone turnover.
- Common sites include pelvis, skull, vertebrae, femurs and tibias.
- Symptoms include bone or joint pain, increased warmth over bone, fracture, bone deformity, syndromes of neural compression.
- Development of an osteogenic sarcoma is a very rare but usually fatal complication.

Skull

- Increased skull size with frontal bossing, calvarial ridging
- Common: hearing loss, increased warmth over skull, headache
- Rare: cranial nerve palsies, hydrocephalus from basilar invagination and CSF flow blockage, vision loss

Pelvis

- Deformity of pelvic bones
- Achiness across sacrum, pelvic ilia, or ischia
- Acetabular deformity with secondary osteoarthritis of the hip

Vertebrae

- Back pain
- Spinal deformity (kyphosis, forward tilt, scoliosis)
- Lumbar radiculopathy and/or spinal stenosis
- Vertebral enlargement, compression fracture
- Rarely, thoracic level spinal cord compression

Extremities

- Bone pain
- Bowing deformity with leg length inequality, gait abnormality
- Secondary osteoarthritis of joints adjacent to bowed limb
- Bone enlargement
- Warmth over affected tibia
- Susceptibility to fracture, especially with advancing osteolytic disease (e.g., "blade of grass" lesion)

Indications for Medical Treatment

- Treat symptoms likely to be due to the pagetic process and likely to respond to a decrease in the increased bone turnover.
  - Examples: pain, increased warmth, some joint and neural compression symptoms
- Treat asymptomatic cases to prevent future complications if disease is biochemically active and present where progression may lead to bone deformity, secondary arthritis, neural compression, or fracture.
  - Examples: asymptomatic involvement of skull (extensive), vertebrae, weight-bearing extremity, acetabular region of pelvis

Specific Anti-Pagetic (Anti-Osteoclast) Therapy in the United States

- Approved therapies:
  - Bisphosphonates: etidronate, pamidronate, alendronate, tiludronate, risedronate
  - Salmon calcitonin
- Available but not approved for Paget's disease:
  - Plicamycin
  - Gallium nitrate
  - Intranasal salmon calcitonin
- Investigational only (for Paget's disease):
  - Bisphosphonates: zoledronate, ibandronate

Treatment with Etidronate

- Etidronate is sold as Didronel
- Dose and duration: 5mg/kg/day orally (400 mg in most patients) for 6 months, followed by at least 6 months off therapy
- Repeated 6 months on/6 month off cycles may be repeated for several years with maintenance of benefit in some, partial loss of effect in others
- Symptom relief often seen after 2–3 months; 50% suppression of SAP at 6 months typical
- Dose given once daily midway in a four hour fast (e.g., between meals) or QHS if no food prior two hours
- No effect on serum calcium; serum phosphate may increase 1 mg/dl

Etidronate Adverse Effects

- Diarrhea (uncommon), mild transient increase in bone pain
- Osteolytic disease in a weight-bearing bone is a contraindiction, as lytic disease may progress with etidronate.
- Doses in excess of recommended amounts and/or longer than recommended duration without appropriate off-drug interval may cause focal osteomalacia with risk of increased bone pain and/or fracture.

Treatment with Pamidronate

- Pamidronate is sold as Aredia
- Package insert recommends 30 mg IV daily for three days, each given as a four-hour infusion in 500 cc normal saline or 5% dextrose in water
- Alternative dosing: individualize dosing to the patient, with goal of normal or near normal serum alkaline phosphatase
  - Mild disease, e.g., serum alkaline phosphatase < 2–3 times upper limit of normal: give one or two 60 mg infusions a few days to one to two weeks apart; check serum alkaline phosphatase 6–8 weeks later; normal or near normal SAP likely, often lasting up to a year; monitor lab every 6 months and re-treat when elevated again
  - Moderate to severe disease, e.g., SAP >3–4 times upper limit of normal: give three to four 60 mg infusions weekly (patient and MD convenience) with check of SAP 6 weeks after last dose; give additional infusions after this if SAP still significantly above normal; follow SAP every 4 to 6 months; avoid more than 600 mg in 12 months
- Provide daily calcium intake of 1000–1500 mg and vitamin D of 400 IU daily to avoid hypocalcemia in early weeks after treatment

Pamidronate Adverse Effects

- About 30% of patients develop one day of fever, myalgias, transient lympho/ leukopenia ("Aredia flu") after first infusion, with symptoms responsive to analgesics/ antipyretics.
- Hypophosphatemia (mild); hypocalcemia (if not on adequate intake)
- Rare iritis, uveitis (responsive to topical steroids)
- Local venous irritation if inadequate fluid volume given

Treatment with Alendronate

- Alendronate is sold as Fosamax
- Dose and duration: 40 mg daily for 6 months; in the clinical trials this led to an average 80% fall in SAP, with normalization of SAP in over 60% of subjects; pain relief after 2–3 months
- Re-treatment guidelines not yet clear, but re-treatment 6 or more months after end of initial treatment if SAP increases significantly above nadir has been suggested
- Dose given upon arising in the AM with 8 oz. tap water, no other PO intake and no lying down for 30 minutes after the dose
- Calcium intake 1000–1500 mg and vitamin D 400 IU daily required during treatment
- Monitor SAP, serum calcium and phosphate every 3 months on drug, and at 4–6 month intervals thereafter

Alendronate Adverse Effects

- GI upset possible in a minority of patients (upper abdominal pain, nausea, dyspepsia, or diarrhea)
- Hypocalcemia, hypophosphatemia if intake of calcium and D inadequate
- No evidence of mineralization defects at 40 mg dose

Treatment with Tiludronate

- Tiludronate is sold as Skelid
- Dose and duration: 400 mg (two 200 mg tablets taken together) daily for 3 months; in the clinical trials this led to an average 50–60% fall in SAP by the end of the 3 months in more than 60% of subjects, with a slight further fall by 3 months later.
- Re-treatment recommendations are not yet defined, but a second 3 month course could be given following the initial 3 month treatment and 3 month off treatment follow-up if SAP levels begin to rise.
- Tiludronate should be taken at a time two hours away from meals with 6–8 oz. of plain water only. Calcium supplements, if indicated, must be taken at least two hours before or after tiludoronate.
- Monitor SAP every 3–6 months during and after therapy.

Tiludronate Adverse Effects

- Mild GI upset in a minority of patients, including nausea, diarrhea, dyspepsia
- No evidence of mineralization defects at the 400 mg dose

Treatment with Risedronate

- Risedronate is sold as Actonel
- Dose and duration: 30 mg daily for 2 months; in the clinical trials this led to an 85% fall in SAP, with normalization of the SAP in over 75% of subjects; pain relief after 2–3 months.
- Initial re-treatment can be considered after a two-month posttreatment observation period, with an additional two months of treatment at the 30 mg dose if SAP remains significantly above normal.
- Dose given upon arising in the AM with 8 oz plain water, no other PO intake, and no lying down for 30 minutes after the dose
- Calcium intake 1000–1500 mg and vitamin D 400 IU daily required during treatment
- Monitor SAP, serum calcium, and phosphate before and after treatment, and at 6-month intervals thereafter.

Risedronate Adverse Effects

- GI upset possible in a minority of patients (upper abdominal pain, nausea, dyspepsia, or diarrhea)
- Hypocalcemia, hypophosphatemia if intake of calcium and D inadequate
- No evidence of mineralization defects at 30 mg dose

Treatment with Salmon Calcitonin (SCT)

- SCT sold as Calcimar or Miacalcin
- Dose: initially 100 U SCT by SQ injection once daily
- Duration: symptoms may improve after 3-6 weeks and serum alkaline phosphatase (SAP) usually falls by 50% at 6 months
  - Often dose can be reduced to 50–100 U SCT three times weekly with continued symptom and SAP benefit for several years in some patients.

Calcitonin Adverse Effects and Loss of Efficacy

- Nausea common in a significant minority; vomiting, diarrhea less common
- Flushing of skin of the face, ears and palms may occur shortly after injection, persisting minutes to hours
- Escape from efficacy (SAP rises, symptoms recur) after 2-3 years of treatment in some patients due to neutralizing antibodies or down regulation of receptors on osteoclasts

Other Treatment Modalities

- Analgesics and NSAIDs helpful for pain symptoms from bone or adjacent joints
- Walking aids, shoe lifts, canes, physical therapy for gait problems due to bowing of leg(s)
- Orthopedic intervention for fracture, impending fracture, joint replacement, osteotomy
- Neurosurgical intervention for spinal stenosis, refractory radiculopathy, hydrocephalus
- Always attempt pretreatment with anti-pagetic therapy (especially pamidronate) prior to elective surgery on pagetic bone to minimize blood loss

Costs of Anti-Pagetic Treatment

- Etidronate 400 mg: $4 per tablet, $120 per month times 6 months
- Pamidronate 60 mg: $300–400 for 60 mg, plus infusion costs
- Alendronate 40 mg: $4 per tablet, $120 per month times 6 months
- Tiludronate 400 mg: with patient rebate plan, about $235 per month for 3 months
- Risedronate 30 mg: $750 to $800 for a 2-month course
- Salmon calcitonin injectable: between $250 and $375 per month for 100 U daily
- Salmon calcitonin nasal spray: 200 IU, $50 per month (off label use)

Resource

The Paget Foundation for Paget's Disease of Bone and Related Disorders, 120 Wall Street, New York, NY 10005.

References

1. Kanis JA. Pathophysiology and treatment of Paget's disease of bone. 2nd Ed. London: Martin Dunitz, 1998.

2. Siris ES. Clinical review: Paget's disease of bone. *J Bone Miner Res* 1998;13:1061–1065.

26

Renal Bone Diseases

Jack W. Coburn

Types and Classification

- High/normal bone turnover (excess PTH)
  - Mild hyperparathyroidism
  - Osteitis fibrosa
- Low bone turnover
  - Aluminum toxicity: osteomalacia or aplastic bone
  - Adynamic bone without Al^{+++} (oversuppressed PTH)
- Mixed bone disease: features of both
  - May represent transition from "low" to "high" turnover
- Dialysis amyloidosis (not "metabolic bone disease" but symptoms mimic other disorders)

Background

Major Role of Kidney in Mineral Homeostasis

- Regulation of serum calcium
  - Calcium-receptor on renal tubules (in common with parathyroid glands and calcitonin-secreting C-cells of thyroid): regulates serum Ca; increased urine Ca allows for escape from hypercalcemia
  - Source of synthesis of circulating calcitriol
    - Target for PTH actions to enhance Ca-reabsorption and to stimulate calcitriol synthesis
  - Site of $24,25(OH)_2D_3$ action to reduce calcitriol synthesis
  - Site of action of calcitriol to stimulate calbindin production
- Regulation of serum phosphorus
  - Target of PTH action to reduce PO_4-reabsorption
  - Permits for excretion of P following its intestinal absorption or its release by tissue catabolism
  - Site of phosphate effect on calcitriol synthesis
  - Site for conservation of P in face PO_4-restriction

- Regulation of serum magnesium
  - Site of excretion of Mg absorbed via intestine with Ca-receptor controlling tubular Mg-reabsorption
  - Site of Mg-retention during Mg-deprivation (? involves Ca-receptor)
- Other
  - Site of degradation of PTH fragments; serum levels of carboxy-terminal PTH and mid-region PTH are increased due to their retention with renal failure

From these many interactions, it is apparent why mineral homeostasis is affected with failure of renal function.

2° Hyperparathyroidism

Pathogenic Factors
- Phosphate retention (hyperphosphatemia)
- Hypocalcemia (low ionized calcium)
  - Reduced renal synthesis of calcitriol
  - Loss of nephron mass—metabolic acidosis
  - Altered transtubular phosphate transport
- Altered parathyroid synthesis/secretion:
  - Reduced calcitriol synthesis
  - Reduced expression of $1,25(OH)_2D$ receptor
  - Change in "set point"
  - Parathyroid hyperplasia: diffuse/nodular
- Resistance to PTH action: bone, other tissues
- Metabolic acidosis

Clinical Features
- No symptoms: most common, symptoms develop with time and greater severity; physical exam: negative
- Bone pain: shoulders, hands, hips, knees; usually aggravated by activity, weight-bearing
- Proximal muscle weakness: insidious onset, often ignored by patient and doctor until crutches are needed
- Pruritus: not specific, many other causes in uremia
- Hypercalcemia: with or without symptoms, pruritus
- Spontaneous tendon rupture: quadriceps, pateller and other tendons; occur with minimal trauma
- Bony deformities: common in children (slipped epiphyses, bowing of long bones; adults can get funnel chest, etc.)
- Fractures: not very common
- Calciphylaxis: vascular calcifications and cutaneous necrosis

Bone Biopsy Features in Trabecular Bone

- Osteitis fibrosa (in trabecular bone)
  - Excess peritrabecular fibrosis (reason for the name)
  - Elevated bone formation rate determined from "double tetracycline labelling"
  - Increased rows of active osteoblasts over unmineralized osteoid
  - Increased osteoclast number overlying eroded surface
  - Increased eroded surface (Howship's lacunae, inactive)
  - Woven osteoid fibrils that contrast to the lamellar pattern in normal bone
- Mild hyperparathyroid bone disease
  - Pertrabecular fibrosis minimally increased
  - Some of above features with bone formation above normal or within the normal range

Laboratory and Radiographic Features

- Laboratory features
  - Elevated intact PTH: usually > 3–5-fold normal
  - Hypercalcemia, particulary when serum P is reduced
  - Hyperphosphatemia: common in all ESRD patients, Often more marked as PO_4 arises partly from bone
  - Elevated alkaline phosphatase: common but not invariable, particularly after vitamin D Rx.
  - Osteocalcin: less specific than PTH; levels elevated in all renal failure patients
  - Anemia that responds poorly to erythropoetin
- Radiographic abnormalities: often minimal or absent
  - Subperiosteal erosions: evident on radial surfaces of digits, distal clavicle, about pelvis
  - Osteosclerosis: most common in thoracic and lumbar vertebrae
  - Brown tumors: quite rare in renal 2° hyperparathyroidism
  - Granular, mottled appearance of skull
  - Periarticular and tumoral calcifications (nonspecific)
  - Vascular calcifications often present but nonspecific

Diagnosis and Treatment

- Diagnosis
  - There is spectrum from mild to severe
  - Serum intact PTH is most useful, particularly in patients without hypercalcemia and not on vitamin D
  - Alkaline phosphatase: progressive increase with time; normal glutamyl transferase excludes liver sources; variable, particularly after vitamin D Rx
  - Bone biopsy: needed only when aluminum toxicity must be excluded, particularly before parathyroid surgery
  - Presence of symptoms implies severe disease

- Treatment
  - Control hyperphosphatemia (often difficult) but essential *before* vitamin D is given
  - Treat hypocalcemia: usually resolves as serum P falls
  - Calcitriol therapy: Initiate Rx after serum P is lowered
  - Parathyroidectomy: necessary when hypercalcemia exists and/or hyperphosphatemia precludes the effective action of vitamin D to reduce serum iPTH appropriately; urgent when calciphylaxis is present
  - If Al-loading coexists, it should be treated *first.*

Therapeutic Considerations

- Control of hyperphosphatemia: serum P, 4–6 mg/dl
  - 1. Dietary P restriction: <1000 mg/day
  - 2. Phosphate binders: $CaCO_3$/CaAcetate, with doses adjusted to reduce serum P
  - 3. Adequate dialysis: P removal
    All 3 are needed
- Maintaining proper serum Ca
  - Choosing proper dialysate Ca
  - With Ca-based binders, lower D-Ca useful
- Reduction of high serum PTH levels
  - Calcitriol therapy: oral/IV
  - Future: calcimimetic agents acting on Ca-receptor; "safer" vitamin D compounds
  - Avoid "oversuppression" of PTH:
    - target for intact PTH: 150–250 pg/ml

Treatment/Prevention in "Early" Renal Failure

- Progression of chronic renal failure (CRF)
  - Most patients progress from mild to advanced renal failure.
  - When GFR is subnormal by 40–50%, altered PO_4 homeostasis, elevated iPTH levels, and lower calcitriol levels are found.
  - Consider results of "treating" such 2° hyperparathyroidism
- Dietary phosphate restriction (low PO_4 diet and/or PO_4-binders)
  - Serum iPTH falls
  - Serum calcitriol rises with GFR >40 but not with worse renal failure
- Calcitriol therapy (daily; doses, 0.125 to 0.5 μg/day)
  - Serum Ca rises slightly
  - Serum P unchanged or even falls slightly.
  - Serum PTH falls and bone biopsies improve toward normal.
  - GFR not affected differently during calcitriol than placebo.
- Conclusion: PO_4-restriction and/or low dose calcitriol therapy should be considered in patients with high serum iPTH or those at "high" risk: all children, females > males, those with slowly progressive disease, tubulointerstitial diseases, and younger patients.

Aluminum Toxicity

Biology of Aluminum

- Ubiquitous in nature: highly insoluble in most forms
- Solubility increases as pH is lowered or raised
  - "Acid rain" may increase its solubility
- Very poor intestinal absorption (<0.1%)
  - Citrate salts *markedly* enhance absorption
- In serum, Al^{+++} is highly protein-bound(>90%)
  - Most bound to transferrin, which may lead to its specific tissue deposition
- Kidneys account for almost all excretion of body Al^{+++}
  - Renal failure major risk factor for Al-toxicity.
- Body distribution: lungs (in macrophages from dust) >bone > liver> respiratory system > kidney> CNS

Sources of Aluminum Loading

- Dialysate: (hemodialysate or peritoneal dialysate)
- Ingestion of aluminum-containing gels
- Other aluminum-containing drugs: e.g., sucrafate (Carafate)
- Parenteral fluids/drugs: e.g., albumin solutions, TPN solutions
- Ingestion of citrate salts: markedly enhances aluminum absorption
- Unidentified sources

Clinical Features and Syndromes Encountered

- Aluminum-related bone disease
  - Osteomalacia or aplastic disease (usually symptomatic)
  - Epidemic form: high dialysate Al; appears quickly and is associated with encephalopathy and anemia
  - Endemic form: from Al-gel ingestion; appears slowly; encephalopathy and microcytic anemia are rare
- Proximal myopathy: often associated with Al-bone disease
- Dialysis encephalopathy: insidious and slowly progressive in patients with "moderate" Al loading
- Acute aluminum neurotoxicity: abrupt onset, seizures, obtundation, myoclonus, coma, and death; factors are very high dialysate Al, oral Al plus citrate or deferoxamine Rx
- Microcytic anemia (with normal Fe): more common in patients with Al-contaminated dialysate

Adverse Effects of Aluminum on Bone

- Direct inhibition of mineralization:
  - Inhibits calcium-phosphate crystal formation
  - Inhibits maturation: Ca-phosphate to hydroxyapatite
- Impaired activity of osteoblasts
- Reduced secretion of PTH
  - Direct effect on parathyroid gland
  - Via the effect of hypercalcemia
- Impaired synthesis of $1,25(OH)_2D_3$
  - Probably not significant in ESRD

Thus, aluminum's adverse effect on bone formation is not surprising

Features and Diagnosis

- Clinical features: can be severe; debilitating bone pain, fractures, and proximal muscle weakness
- Laboratory and radiographic features
  - Hypercalcemia common, often when the dialysate Ca >3.0 mEq/l and/or $CaCO_3$/CaAcetate as P-binders
  - Serum iPTH: usually below 100–150 pg/ml, but 10–15% of Al-loaded patients have iPTH >200 pg/ml.
  - Serum Al: often >75 µg/L, but can be <50 µg/L if there has been no Al exposure for > 4–6 months.
  - X-rays: often show demineralization; undisplaced pseudofractures may detected only by scintiscan.
- Diagnosis: most important if parathyroid surgery is contemplated and there is history of Al exposure.
  - DFO infusion test: serum Al increment >100 µg/L after DFO, 40 mg/kg, or rise >50 µg/L after 5 mg/kg provide presumptive evidence of Al loading
  - Bone biopsy remains the "gold standard" for the diagnosis.

Management

- Prevention is much preferred to treatment
  - Avoid use of Al-containing phosphate-binders
  - Proper H_2O purification for dialysate preparation
  - Avoid citrate intake in ESRD patients unless Al-intake is vigorously avoided
- Total withdrawal of exposure to Al^{+++} as therapy
  - No Al-gels as P-binders (use $CaCO_3$/CaAcetate) *and* Dialysate Al <5µg/L: Al-bone disease improves
- Deferoxamine (Desferal or DFO) treatment
  - DFO chelates Al and augments dialysis Al-removal, *but* it enhances the risk of fatal mucormycosis.
  - Limit DFO-treatment to Al-neurotoxicity which is not improved after total withdrawal of Al-exposure.
  - Low DFO dose: 5 mg/kg given every 9–10 days

Interactions with Parathyroid Hormone

- Aluminum localizes in the parathyroid gland
- Al^{+++} can inhibit PTH secretion (in vivo and in vitro)
- ESRD patients with very high PTH levels
  - Al-bone disease is infrequent despite Al loading
  - Diffuse Al localization in bone rather than on surface
- In Al-loaded patient having parathyroidectomy: Al-bone disease either worsens or appears de novo, even without additional Al loading
- PTH injections into Al-loaded rats results in greater bone Al than Al loading without PTH.

Low Bone Turnover State

"Aplastic/Adynamic" Bone—Is It a Disease?

- Bone biopsy: low bone formation; No Al^{+++}
  - Reduced numbers of osteoblasts/osteoclasts

Risk Factor: ? Oversuppressed PTH

- Use of $CaCO_3$/CaAcetate as PO_4-binders
- CAPD with use of dialysate Ca >3.0 mEq/liter
- Diabetes mellitus/older patients
- Intact PTH <100–150 pg/ml (Normal, 15–65)

Features

- No signs/symptoms
- Risk of hypercalcemia with use of CaSalt or vit D; greater risk of Al-toxicity with use of Al-gels?
- Higher fracture risk after renal transplant

Diagnosis and Management

- Diagnosis
  - Aluminum loading must be excluded.
  - By definition, this is a bone biopsy diagnosis. A biopsy is rarely needed unless hypercalcemia is a major diagnostic and therapeutic problem.
  - Serum iPTH levels <100 pg/mI strongly support the diagnosis and iPTH <150 pg/ml are suggestive.
  - Background: older age, use of $CaCO_3$/CaAcetate, short duration of dialysis, calcitriol therapy with iPTH <200 pg/ml, and/or no exposure to Al
- Management
  - In asymptomatic patients, no treatment needed
    - Avoid use of aluminum gels
    - Avoid use of calcitriol
    - Consider reducing dialysate Ca concentration

Intact PTH levels in End-Stage Renal Disease

Approximate IPTH Range with Bone Disorders

Disorder	Intact PTH*
• Hyperparathyroidism	
– Mild	200–400
– Moderate	350–800
– Severe	>700
• Aluminum Bone Disease	10–500
	Most <100
• Aplastic/adynamic bone	<100–150

*Normal, 10–65 pg/ml. Exceptions: presence of hypercalcemia; prolonged vitamin D Rx

Hypercalcemia

Causes in End-stage Renal Disease

• 2° Hyperparathyroidism	• Dialysate Ca >3.0 mEq/liter*
• Aluminum-bone disease	• Marked hypophosphatemia
• Low BFR (adynamic bone)	• Calcitriol synthesis (sarcoid, Tbc, etc.)
• $CaCO_3$/CaAcetate therapy*	• Malignancy (PTHrP)
• Calcitriol therapy*	• Immobilization*

*Often coexisting/precipitating factor

Dialysis Amyloidosis

Definition and Clinical Features

- Unique amyloid comprised of β-2 microglobulin
  - Deposited in tendons, bone, periarticular structures
- Carpal tunnel syndrome: most common manifestation
- Pain: shoulder, hands, hips, knees, neck
  - Nocturnal, partially relieved by activity
  - Analgesics are largely ineffective
- Destructive cervical spondyloarthropathy
- Multiple thin-walled bone cysts at ends of long bones—wrists, shoulders, femurs
- Camptodactyly, trigger fingers
- Tendon cysts and synovitis
- Hip fractures

Diagnosis and Management

- Diagnosis
  - Clinical features of carpal tunnel syndrome (CTS) and scapulohumoral pain that is worse with rest combined with multiple thin-walled cysts in upper humerus, hip, and metacarpals permit the clinical diagnosis.
  - Bone cysts often misdiagnosed as "brown tumors."
  - Background: appears after 5–10 years of hemodialysis, symptoms and features appear sooner in those starting dialysis after age 50. Unheard of in children.
- Management
  - Largely unsatisfactory
  - Surgery for CTS highly useful; late recurrence is common.
  - Microsynovectomy for certain tendons of the hands
  - Steroid injections in affected joints: shoulders, hips
  - NSAIDs may ease symptoms.
  - Renal transplantation: pain disappears, but amyloid deposits of β-2 microglobulin remain unchanged.
  - "High flux" hemodialysis may slow the clinical appearance.

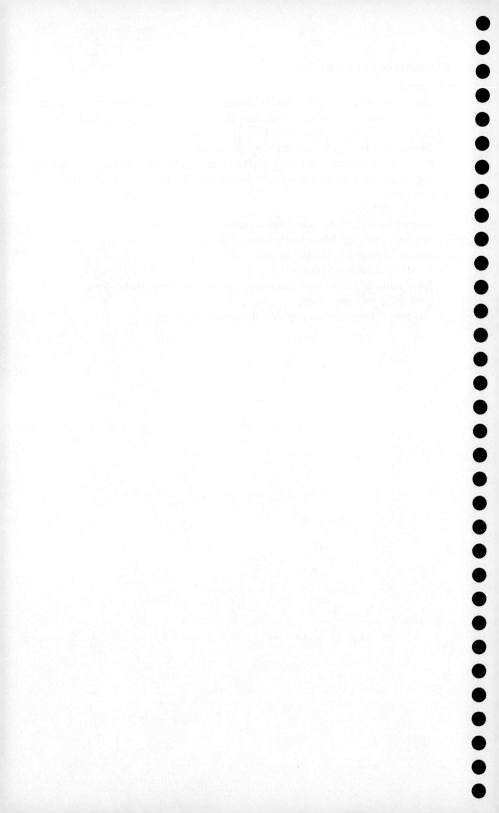

27

Metastatic Bone Disease

Robert F. Gagel

Bone Metastasis

- 25% of cancer patients who die have bone metastasis
  - Metastasis is most common in
    - breast—75%
    - lung—35%
    - kidney—25%
    - gastrointestinal, thyroid, pancreatic, ovarian—10–15%
  - Metastasis most commonly located
    - vertebrae—75%
    - pelvis—40%
    - femur—25%
    - skull and upper extremities—10–15%

Clinical Characteristics

- Localized pain—intermittent and unrelated to activity
- Shoulder girdle metastasis—frozen shoulder
- Secondary epidural compression from vertebral metastasis
  - Increasing back pain
- Pathologic fracture

Diagnosis of Bone Metastasis

- Radiographic
  - Standard x-rays and bone scan
  - Magnetic resonance imaging
    - sensitive screen for bone metastasis, expecially vertebral

The Bone and Mineral Manual
Copyright ©1999 by Academic Press

- Laboratory evaluation
  - Serum calcium mandatory to exclude hypercalcemia
  - Optional but useful markers of bone turnover
    - serum alkaline phosphatase
    - serum osteocalcin
    - urine collagen degradation products: deoxypyridinoline crosslinks, NTX
- Fine needle aspiration
  - Indications
    - document metastasis in single suspicious radiographic lesion
    - obtain tissue for special studies
  - A solitary lesion may be primary tumor or metastatic lesion

Therapeutic Options for Bone Metastasis

- Prevention
  Monthly pamidronate in breast carcinoma
- Treatment
  - Immediate internal fixation for long bone fracture
  - X-ray therapy
    - 2000–5000 cGy for pain relief
    - 5000–7000 cGy—reossification in 75%
    - balance marrow suppression vs. tumor growth
  - Radionuclides
    - radioactive iodine—thyroid carcinoma
    - strontium 35
    - radioiodinated bisphosphonates
  - Surgical excision of isolated metastasis in occasional cases
  - Adequate analgesia
    - x-ray therapy
    - opioids
    - local nerve blocks

For evaluation and management of hypercalcemia complicating metastatic bone disease, see Chapter 31.

28

Osteomalacia

John G. Haddad, Jr.*
Ethel S. Siris

Definition

- Failure to deposit the inorganic mineral phase in the newly formed organic bone matrix of adults
- A decreased mineralization rate, and often a decrease in staining intensity and the extent of the mineralization front are detected by histomorphometry of a bone biopsy specimen.

Pathogenetic Mechanisms

- Hypophosphatemia
  - leads to low concentrations of inorganic phosphorus at sites of mineralization
  - decreased Ca/P product (<30 mg/dl) often found; rarely, a low calcium with normal to high phosphorus (hypoparathyroidism) can cause condition
- Acidosis
  - decreased hydroxyapatite synthesis and bone mineralization when body pH is lower than normal
- Hyphophosphatasia
  - poor alkaline phosphatase activity leads to decreased hydrolysis of inorganic pyrophosphate (mineralization inhibitor).
- Fibrogenesis imperfecta ossium
  - abnormal bone matrix leads to its hypomineralization.
- Drug
  - high dose, protracted administration of some bisphosphonate compounds can interfere with matrix mineralization.

Types

Vitamin D Deficiency

- Inadequate solar exposure, malabsorption, poor intake, nephrotic syndromes

*Deceased

The Bone and Mineral Manual
Copyright ©1999 by Academic Press
All rights of reproduction in any form reserved.

Disorders of Vitamin D Metabolism

- Inadequate 25(OH) vitamin D 1α-hydroxylation
  - Renal diseases, failure; tumor-associated osteomalacia
  - Genetic (vitamin D-dependent rickets Type I, X-linked hypophosphatemia)
- Accelerated vitamin D and 25(OH) vitamin D catabolism
  - Drugs (anti-convulsants)
  - Calcium deficiency; $1,25(OH)_2D$ administration
- Resistance to $1,25(OH)_2D$
  - Genetic (vitamin D-dependent rickets Type II)
  - Intestinal diseases, resections

Acidosis

- Distal renal tubular acidosis
  - Primary (sporadic, familial)
  - Secondary (galactosemia, Fabry's disease)
- Hypergammaglobulinemic states
- Medullary sponge kidney
- Following renal transplantation and enteral bladder constructs
- Drugs (acetazolamide, chemotherapy, $NH_4Cl.$)
- Chronic renal disease

Renal Tubular Disorders (Fanconi's Syndrome)

- Associated with systemic process (cystinosis, Lowe's, glycogenosis)
- Primary renal (idiopathic, sporadic, familial)
- Systemic diseases
  - Hereditary (Wilson's disease, tyrosinemia)
  - Acquired (myeloma, nephrotic syndrome, renal transplants)
- Toxins (cadmium, lead, "old" tetracycline)

Phosphate Depletion

- Dietary (low intake, aluminum hydroxide antacids)
- Tumor-associated ("oncogenic") osteomalacia
- X-linked hypophosphatemia
- Hypophosphatemia/hypercalciuria osteomalacia
- Sporadic phosphate diabetes

Defective Matrix Synthesis

- Hypophosphatasia
- Fibrogenesis imperfecta ossium
- Aluminum intoxication

Defective Matrix Mineralization

- Some bisphosphonates (primarily etidronate)
- NaF (rapid matrix synthesis outpaces mineralization)

Findings that Suggest Adult Calciferol Deficiency

Clinical

- Marginal calciferol intake
- Malabsorption, anti-convulsant medications
- Little/no sunshine exposure
- Variable limb, rib, pelvic pain/tenderness
- Proximal myopathy

Laboratory

- Persistent hypophosphatemia
- Decreased serum calcium-phosphate product (<30 mg/dl)
- Decreased urine calcium excretion (<75 mg/24 hrs)
- Decreased serum 25(OH) vitamin D (<10 ng/ml)
- Increased serum PTH
- Increased serum alkaline phosphatase (bone)
- Decreased serum HCO_3^-
- Increased serum Cl^-
- Increased urine excretion of bone Type I collagen degradation products
- Increased serum osteocalcin

Radiology

- Subperiosteal resorption
- Cortical tunneling
- Coarsened trabeculae
- Pseudofractures (Looser zones)

Features of Phosphate Wasting

Dietary, Aluminum Binding

- 2° renal conservation of phosphorus (?mediator)
- Ca/P egress from bone (failed mineralization)
- 2° hypoparathyroidism—hypercalciuria
- Reversal with normal intestinal phosphorus absorption

Renal Phosphate Wasting

- Low serum inorganic phosphate
- Insufficient $1,25(OH)_2D$ production (XLH)
- Inappropriate renal conservation of phosphorus
- Low Ca/P product $\rightarrow$ poor skeletal mineralization

Oncogenic Phosphaturia

- Tumor secretes phosphaturic humor
- Tumor product suppresses $1,25(OH)_2D$ production
- Low serum inorganic phosphate
- Low Ca/P product $\rightarrow$ poor skeletal mineralization
- Reversal with tumor excision

Features of Acidosis

Kidney Fails to Excrete Protons

- Urine pH>5 after NH_4Cl loading
- Hypercalciuria often (poor skeletal deposition of Ca/P)—early
- Systemic acidosis depresses intestinal calcium absorption
- 2° HPT with renal losses and intestinal malabsorption of calcium—late
- 2° HPT hypophosphatemia

Acidosis and Other Tubular Dysfunctions

- Phosphate wasting—primary
- Renal calcium leak
- Decreased $1,25(OH)_2D$ production
- 2° HPT with renal losses and intestinal malabsorption of calcium

Laboratory Screening

Total Serum Calcium

- Normal (early vitamin D deficiency)
- Low (late vitamin D deficiency, resistance)
- High (1° HPT)

Total Serum Phosphate

- Low (XLH, Fanconi; 1° and 2° HPT; oncogenic)
- High (CRF)

Urine Calcium

- Low (malabsorption, vitamin D deficiency; CRF)
- Normal (XLH, RTA-late)
- High (nutritional phosphate wasting; RTA early; hereditary; hypophosphatemic rickets with hypercalciuria)

iPTH

- Low (nutritional wasting; RTA early; hypoparathyroidism)
- Normal (XLH; RTA early; oncogenic; Fanconi)
- High (CRD; 1° HPT; 2° (vitamin D deficiency, malabsorption); vitamin D resistance

Serum Bicarbonate

• Normal (early vitamin D deficiency; 1° and 2° HPT; Fanconi)
• Low (late vitamin D deficiency; 2° HPT; Fanconi)

Serum Alkaline Phosphatase

• Low (hypophosphatasia)
• High (most other syndromes)

Serum 25(OH) Vitamin D

• Low (vitamin D deficiency; malabsorption)
• Normal (most other syndromes)

Serum 1,25(OH)$_2$D

– Low (late vitamin D deficiency; XLH; some Fanconi; CRD; oncogenic; cadmium; hypoparathyroidism)
– Normal (early vitamin D deficiency; Fanconi)
– High (nutritional phosphate depletion; vitamin D receptor mutations; early vitamin D repletion; 1° HPT)

Therapy

Vitamin D Deficiency

• Oral or parenteral vitamin D supplements
• Sunshine exposure
• Correct malabsorption (gluten-free diet)

Disordered Vitamin D Metabolism

• Supplement vitamin D (anticonvulsants, Type I vitamin D dependency)
• Supplement 1,25(OH)$_2$D (CRD; XLH; hypoparathyroidism; some sporadic hypophosphatemias)
• Remove tumor (oncogenic; 1° HPT)
• Remove toxin (cadmium)

Phosphate Wasting

• Supplement phosphate (sodium, potassium phosphate salts to tolerance (diarrhea) in divided doses)
• Reduce 2° HPT (supplement calcium, vitamin D or active vitamin D)

Acidosis

• Add bicarbonate
• Reduce 2° HPT (supplement calcium, vitamin D or active vitamin D)
• Dialysis, renal transplantation

Skeletal Mineralization

- Remove toxin (chelate Al^{+++}; discontinue bisphosphonates; discontinue or decrease NaF administration.

References

1. Bikle DD. Bone disease due to nutritional, gastrointestinal and hepatic disorders. In: Coe FL, Favus MJ, (eds), *Disorders of Bone and Mineral Metabolism*. New York: Raven Press 1992;951–976.

2. Dent CE, and Stamp TCB. Vitamin D, rickets and osteomalacia. In: Avioli LV, Krane SM, (eds), *Metabolic Bone Disease*, New York: Academic Press 1977;237–306.

3. Ericksen EF, Axelrod DW, Melsen F. *Bone Histomorphometry: An Official Publication of ASBMR*. New York: Raven Press 1994;56–58.

4. Finch PJ, Ang L, Eastwood JB, Maxwell JD. Clinical and histological spectrum of osteomalacia among Asians in South London. *Quarterly J Medicine* 1992;83:439–448.

5. Parfitt AM, Rao DS, Stanciu J, et al. Irreversible bone loss in osteomalacia. Comparison of radial photon absorptiometry with iliac bone histomorphometry during treatment. *J Clin Invest* 1985;76:2403–2412.

29

High Bone Mass

Michael P. Whyte

Glossary

Deformity: Alteration in the shape of a previously normal part (e.g., following a fracture)

Dysostosis: Malformation of one or a few individual bones

Dysplasia: Heritable and symmetrical imperfect development of the skeleton

Hyperostosis: Increase in cortical (compact) bone thickness at the periosteal and/or endosteal surface

Malformation: Structural abnormality due to faulty development

Modeling: External shaping of a bone during its growth and development

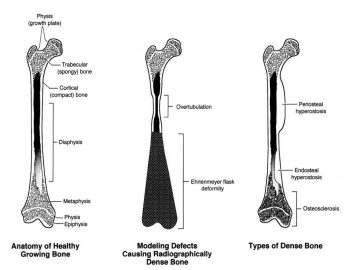

Anatomy of Healthy Growing Bone

Modeling Defects Causing Radiographically Dense Bone

Types of Dense Bone

The Bone and Mineral Manual
Copyright ©1999 by Academic Press
All rights of reproduction in any form reserved.

Physis: Growth plate

Sclerosis: Increased density of trabecular (spongy) bone

Tubulation: Formation of a tube-shaped bone

Disorders That Cause High Bone Mass

Dysplasias and Dysostoses

- Autosomal dominant osteosclerosis
- Central osteosclerosis with ectodermal dysplasia
- Craniodiaphyseal dysplasia
- Craniometaphyseal dysplasia
- Dysosteosclerosis
- Endosteal hyperostosis
  - van Buchem disease
  - Sclerosteosis
- Frontometaphyseal dysplasia
- Infantile cortical hyperostosis (Caffey disease)
- Lenz-Majewski syndrome
- Melorheostosis
- Metaphyseal dysplasia (Pyle disease)
- Mixed-sclerosing, bone dystrophy
- Oculodento-osseous dysplasia
- Osteodysplasia of Melnick and Needles
- Osteoectasia with hyperphosphatasia (hyperostosis corticalis)
- Osteomesopyknosis
- Osteopathia striata
- Osteopetrosis
- Osteopoikilosis
- Pachydermoperiostosis
- Progressive diaphyseal dysplasia (Engelmann disease)
- Pycnodysostosis
- Tubular stenosis (Kenny-Caffey syndrome)

Metabolic Disorders

- Carbonic anhydrase II deficiency
- Fluorosis
- Heavy metal poisoning
- Hepatitis C-associated osteosclerosis
- Hypervitaminosis A, D
- Hyperparathyroidism, hypoparathyroidism, and pseudohypoparathyroidism
- Milk-alkali syndrome
- Renal osteodystrophy
- X-linked hypophosphatemia

Other Disorders

- Axial osteomalacia
- Diffuse idiopathic skeletal hyperostosis (DISH)
- Fibrogenesis imperfecta ossium
- Hypertrophic osteoarthropathy
- Ionizing radiation
- Leukemia
- Lymphoma
- Mastocytosis
- Multiple myeloma
- Myelofibrosis
- Osteomyelitis
- Osteonecrosis
- Paget's disease
- Polycythemia vera
- Sarcoidosis
- Sickle cell disease
- Skeletal metastases
- Tuberous sclerosis

Radiographic Patterns of High Bone Mass

Cortical and Trabecular Bone (Both)

- Carbonic anhydrase II deficiency
- Dysosteosclerosis
- Lenz-Majewski syndrome
- Hepatitis C-associated osteosclerosis
- Osteopetrosis
- Pycnodysostosis

Cortical Bone (Predominantly)

- Autosomal dominant osteosclerosis
- Diffuse idiopathic skeletal hyperostosis (DISH)
- Endosteal hyperostosis
  - Sclerosteosis
  - van Buchem disease
- Hypertrophic osteoarthropathy
- Pachydermoperiostosis
- Progressive diaphyseal dysplasia (Engelmann disease)

Trabecular Bone (Predominantly)

- Dysplastic
  - Central osteosclerosis with ectodermal dysplasia
  - Osteomesopyknosis
- Hematological disorders
  - Mastocytosis
  - Myelofibrosis
  - Polycythemia vera
  - Sickle cell disease
- Metabolic disorders
  - Fluorosis
  - Hyperparathyroidism
  - Renal osteodystrophy
  - X-linked hypophosphatemia
  - Vitamin D toxicity
- Neoplastic Disorders
  - Metastatic disease
  - Myeloma, lymphoma, leukemia

Material in this chapter updated from: Whyte MP. Skeletal Disorders Characterized By Osteosclerosis or Hyperostosis. Avioli LV, Krane SM, (eds), *Metabolic Bone Disease*, 3rd Ed. New York: Academic Press 1998;697–738.

30

Primary Hyperparathyroidism

John P. Bilezikian

General Points

- **Definition:** Incompletely regulated, excessive secretion of parathyroid hormone.
- **Diagnosis:** Elevated serum calcium concentration with concomitant elevation of parathyroid hormone.
- **Cause:** Unknown, but increasingly, molecular defects in the parathyroid hormone gene are being discovered.
- **Incidence:** 1/1000 in the adult population. Female/male ratio 3:1.
- Most patients are discovered without classical signs and symptoms (overt bone and stone disease).
- They are said to be asymptomatic.
- The serum calcium is usually less than 12 mg/dl (NL: 8.4–10.2 mg/dl).
- Parathyroid hormone is usually 25–100% above normal. For the intact parathyroid hormone assay (IRMA), the level is usually between 75 and 130 pg/ml (NL: 10–65).

Role of Bone Mass Measurement

- Noninvasive approaches to bone mass measurement (i.e., dual energy x-ray absorptiometry) often show a reduction in bone density, particularly of cortical bone (i.e., distal 1/3 of the radius).
- It is important to use bone mass measurement to evaluate primary hyperparathyroidism. It is the only noninvasive way to detect early bone involvement in asymptomatic patients.

Surgical Guidelines

- Serum calcium greater than 12 mg/dl
- Urine calcium greater than 400 mg/24 hours
- Presence or history of kidney stones
- Bone density greater than 2 standard deviations below expected for age and sex-matched controls
- Under 50 years of age

The Bone and Mineral Manual
Copyright ©1999 by Academic Press
All rights of reproduction in any form reserved.

Preoperative Localization

• Used most commonly in patients with previous neck surgery
• Sestamibi imaging most accurate and sensitive (75–80%)
• Other noninvasive approaches include ultrasound, MRI, CAT scan

Surgery: Pathology

• In most patients (80%), a single benign adenoma
• In 15–20%, four-gland hyperplasia
• Very rarely (less than 0.5%) a carcinoma

Medical Management

• Avoid dehydration
• Avoid immobilization
• Avoid diuretics
• Keep active
• Keep calcium intake modest

Course

• Patients who do not meet surgical criteria do well with conservative medical
  follow up
• Patients who undergo successful surgery do well
  – Biochemical indices normalize
  – Bone mass increases

31

The Nonparathyroid Chronic and Acute Hypercalcemias

Lawrence E. Mallette

Common Nonparathyroid Hypercalcemias

- Familial benign (hypocalciuric) hypercalcemias
- Malignancy
- $1,25(OH)_2D$ mediated: sarcoidosis
- Milk alkali syndrome (calcium carbonate OTC)
- Thyrotoxicosis

PTH–Mediated Hypercalcemias without Primary Hyperparathyroidism

- Familial benign (hypocalciuric) hypercalcemias (PTH permissive)
  - Inactivating mutation of renal/parathyroid calcium-sensing receptor
- Chronic lithium administration
  - Slow parathyroid enlargement; eventual autonomy or adenoma in some
- Tertiary hyperparathyroidism
  - Autonomous nodules after chronic secondary hyperparathyroidism
- Jansen's metaphyseal dysplasia (very rare)
  - Activating mutation of PTH receptor
- True ectopic PTH production (very rare)

Rare Causes of Nonparathyroid Hypercalcemia

Nonsarcoid Granulomatous Diseases

- Tuberculosis
- Fungal infections (histoplasmosis, coccidiomycosis, cryptococcosis)
- Candidiasis
- Lepromatous leprosy
- Foreign body (silicone) granuloma
- Berylliosis
- Eosinophillic granuloma
- Wegener's granulomatosis
- Granulomatous reaction to malignancy

Medications/Ingestions Causing Hypercalcemia

- Theophylline toxicity
- Lithium toxicity (acute)
- Hypervitaminosis D
- Ingestion of toxic plants (solanum or cestrum)
- Hypervitaminosis A
- Aspirin poisoning
- Thiazide diuretic (potentiates increase from other causes)

Renal/Adrenal/Muscle-Associated

- Adrenocortical insufficiency
- Aluminum intoxication (dialysis or parenteral alimentation)
- Recovery phase after rhabdomyolytic renal failure
- Neuroleptic malignant syndrome

Calcium Overload (Hypercalciuria before Hypercalcemia)

- Immobilization
- Paget's disease with fracture (limb immobilization)
- Near drowning in the Dead Sea
- Variants of milk alkali syndrome
  - Cheese alkalosis syndrome
  - Compulsive chalk eating

Miscellaneous Very Rare Causes

- Sepsis (hypocalcemia is the usual response)
- Massive mammary hyperplasia (PTHrP)
- Williams' syndrome (newborns)
- Pseudohypercalcemia (calcium-binding paraprotein)

Bedside Diagnosis

- Weight loss >20 lbs favors:
  - Malignancy
  - Thyrotoxicosis
  - Addison's disease
  - 1° HPT
- Band keratopathy—rare, usually only in 1° HPT or milk alkali syndrome
- Proximal muscle weakness and hyperreflexla favor
  - 1° HPT
  - Thyrotoxicosis (goiter, tremor, etc.)

Cost-Effective Laboratory Diagnosis

- Begin with intact PTH measurement (plus SPEP, TSH if suspicious)
- Principle: intact PTH normal range is 10 to 65 pg/ml, but hypercalcemia is not normal and should suppress normal parathyroid glands enough to give a PTH value below 25 pg/ml (or below 20 pg/ml if renal function normal).
- If PTH below 25 pg/ml: nonparathyroid hypercalcemia
  - Measure 1,25(OH)$_2$D, SPEP, TSH, 25-hydroxyvitamin D
  - 1,25(OH)$_2$D value above 40 pg/ml granulomatous disease
- If PTH 26-65 pg/ml: parathyroid autonomy
  - Often primary hyperparathyroidism, but . . .
    - consider FBH, lithium, prior secondary hyperparathyroldism
    - consider second contributing cause suppressing PTH (thyroid, thiazide)
- If PTH above 65 pg/ml
  - Primary hyperparathyroidism
  - Occasional FBH or very rare ectopic PTH production
- If PTH value borderline, repeat after serum calcium lowered slightly

Familial Benign Hypercalcemia (FBH)

- Autosomal dominant
  - In 95% of families, a calcium sensing receptor mutation (chromosome 3)
- Hypercalcemia present from birth, relatively stable
- Intact PTH not elevated (97%)
- Normal rise in PTH per unit fall in Ca^{++}, but at a higher Ca^{++} level
- Increased PTH (3%)—usually in older subjects or rarely in a family
- Normal or low urinary calcium (calcium sensing receptor in renal tubule)
- Normal renal phosphate metabolism
- Benign: "no" complications
  - Chief risk: unnecessary parathyroid surgery
  - Transient neonatal hypocalcemia—unaffected infant of FBH mom
  - Severe neonatal hyperparathyroidism—homozygous for FBH receptor(s)

Rational Approach to Excluding FBH

- Check old charts for normal calcium values (excludes congenital hypercalcemia)
- Check serum calcium of both parents (if available)
  - Each sibling or child with normal calcium reduces probability by 50%, but cannot exclude with 100% certainty unless both parents available.
- Urinary Ca/Cr clearance ratio (only if above fail)
  - 24 hour urine collection on no-added-calcium diet
  - Simultaneous blood calcium and creatinine

$$\frac{UCa^{++} \times S\ creatinine}{SCa^{++} \times U\ creatinine}$$

  >13% excludes FBH
  <1.0% c/w FBH, but seen in 5% of 1 HPT

Hypercalcemia of Thyrotoxicosis

- Usually severe hyperthyroidism—increased bone resorption
- Serum phosphate usually high-normal
- Increased alkaline phosphatase common
- PTH suppressed
- Responds to control of hyperthyroidism and possibly to propranolol
- If emergent, treat with calcitonin (pamidronate contraindicted—fever)

Milk Alkali Syndrome

- Originally described from alternating hourly milk and sodium bicarbonate doses
- Calcium carbonate abuse currently the leading cause
- Alkalosis increases GI calcium absorption and renal tubular reabsorption
- Alkalosis predisposes to nephrocalcinosis and renal damage
- Hypercalciuria occurs early, hypercalcemia after GFR has decreased
- Prognosis depends on severity of renal damage

Sarcoidosis

- Unregulated 1-alpha hydroxylation of 25-hydroxyvitamin D by activated macrophages
- Nonsuppressed or increased $1,25(OH)_2D$ causes
  - Increased GI calcium absorption
  - Increased bone resorption
- Untreated sarcoidosis: hypercalciuria in 40–50%, hypercalcemia in 10%
- Serum phosphate usually near upper normal limit or above
- If intact PTH above 25 pg/ml consider concomitant primary hyperparathyroidism.
- Treatment to prevent or treat hypercalcemia
  - Avoidance of sunlight and dietary vitamin D (milk, multivitamins)
  - Low dietary calcium
  - Anti-osteoclast agents (calcitonin, aminobisphosphonates)
  - Hydroxychloroquine lowers $1,25(OH)_2D$—quite effective, bone friendly
  - Glucocorticoids lower $1,25(OH)_2D$

Malignancy–Associated Hypercalcemia

- Most common cause of acute hypercalcemia
- Etiology
  - Production of parathyroid-related peptide (PTHrP) most common
  - Skeletal metastases (may also have increased PTHrP)
  - Myeloma (tumor necrosis factor)
  - Excess calcitriol (1,25 dihydroxyvitamin D)
  - Excess prostaglandin

Treatment of Hypercalcemia—General Principles

- Prevention
  - Avoid immobilization in patients with rapid bone turnover
  - Avoid salt restriction in patients with active or potential hypercalcemia
  - Encourage increased fluid intake and avoidance of dehydration
- Discover and treat underlying cause

Treatment of Emergency Hypercalcemia

- Restore normal blood volume
- Volume expand
- Loop diuretic only after volume expansion
- Hemodialysis/hemofiltration if renal insufficiency
- Use antiresorptive therapy early—to attack source of the excess calcium
  - Pamidronate I.V., 60–90 mg over 4 hours
- High-dose I.V. steroids if hypercalcemia secondary to increased 1,25 dihydroxy-vitamin D (granulomatous diseases, vitamin D intoxication)

References

1. Mallette LE. The hypercalcemias. *Semin Nephrol* 1992;12:159–190.

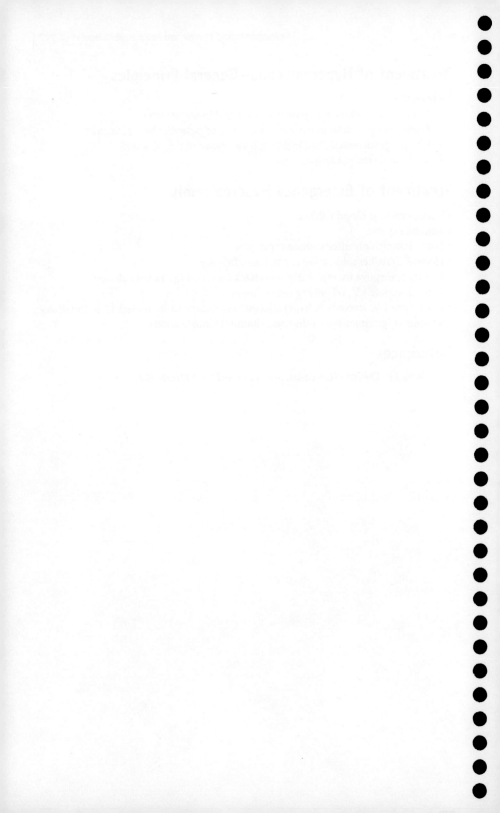

32

Hypocalcemia

Frederick R. Singer

Differential Diagnosis

- Hypoparathyroidism
  - Idiopathic
  - Postoperative
  - Postirradiation
  - Metastatic carcinoma
  - Magnesium deficiency
  - Wilson's disease
  - Hemochromatosis
  - Thalassemia
  - Alcohol
  - DiGeorge (congenital absence of parathyroids)
  - Neonatal
- Parathyroid hormone resistance
  - Pseudohypoparathyroidism Types I and II
  - Renal failure
  - Magnesium deficiency
- Vitamin D deficiency
- Vitamin D-dependent rickets Types I and II
- Acute pancreatitis
- Acute rhabdomyolysis
- Toxic shock syndrome
- Tumor lysis syndrome
- Osteoblastic metasteses
- Postparathyroidectomy (hungry bone syndrome)
- Drug-induced
  - Bisphosphonate, plicamycin, calcitonin, gallium nitrate, phosphate
  - Citrated blood
  - Fluoride excess
  - Foscarnet, pentamidine, ketoconazole
- Prematurity
- Hypoalbuminemia

The Bone and Mineral Manual
Copyright ©1999 by Academic Press
All rights of reproduction in any form reserved.

Signs and Symptoms

Symptoms

- Paresthesias and tingling
- Muscle cramp
- Laryngeal spasm
- Irritability, anxiety, depression
- Seizures

Signs

- Positive Chvostek's sign
- Trousseau's sign
- Prolonged QT interval on ECG
- Delta waves in frontal region of EEG

Therapy

Acute and Subacute

- Intravenous calcium
  - Bolus: 150 mg of calcium gluconate
  - Infusion: 5–10 mg elemental calcium/kg/hour for several hours
  - Parenteral magnesium for magnesium deficient state: 50 mEq Mg/24 hours IV for 5 days

Chronic

- 1000–2000 mg calcium intake divided in 2–3 doses (reduce use of dairy products if serum phosphorus is elevated)
- Pharmacologic doses
  - Vitamin D_2: Average dose 50,000 IU/day or
  - Calcitriol: 0.5–5 µg/day
- Oral magnesium salts for malabsorption or renal magnesium wasting syndromes

Diagnostic Tests

- Serum intact parathyroid hormone
- Serum creatinine and blood urea nitrogen
- Serum 25(OH) vitamin D and 1,25(OH)$_2$ vitamin D
- Serum magnesium
- Urinary cyclic AMP response to parathyroid hormone 1–34

References

1. Eastell R, Heath H III. The hypocalcemic states. Their differential diagnosis and management. In: Coe FL, Favus MJ, (eds), *Disorders of Bone and Mineral Metabolism*. New York: Raven Press 1992;571.

2. Fitzpatrick LA, Arnold A. In: Hypoparathryroidism. De Groot LJ, (ed), *Endocrinology*. 3rd Ed. Philadelphia: W.B. Saunders 1995;1123.

3. Guise TA, Mundy GR. Clinical Review 69: Evaluation of hypocalcemia in children and adults. *J Clin Endocronal Metab* 1985;80:1473.

Part Three

Patient and Family Education and Support

33

Principles of Patient and Family Education and Support

Betsy Love McClung

Patient and Family Education

- Helping patients and their families assume greater responsibility for their own health is a major focus of health education.
- Patients and their families need to work together with health care professionals to establish a partnership to accomplish health care goals.
- Physicians make decisions about therapy.
- Patients make decisions about adherence.
- In order to correctly make decisions, the patient and family members need to know not only what and how, but why, what if, what if not, etc.

Goals of Patient and Family Education

Increase Knowledge and Clarify Misconceptions about Medical Condition

- Definition
- Diagnosis
- Risk factors
- Consequences
- Symptoms
- Treatments
- Prognosis
- Prevention

Implement New Behaviors to Adapt to Medical Condition and Physical Limitations

- Nutrition
- Exercise
- Medications
- Injury prevention
- Pain management

Learn Strategies to Cope with Psychosocial Responses to Disease and Disability

- Anxiety
- Depression
- Anger
- Withdrawal
- Fear

The Bone and Mineral Manual
Copyright ©1999 by Academic Press
All rights of reproduction in any form reserved.

Overcome Barriers to Compliance by Articulating
- Rationale for pharmacologic and nonpharmacologic therapy
- Possible alternatives
- Side effects
- Length of treatment
- How to take
- Reminders
- Ways to simplify

Master Behavior Changes Required to Implement and Continue with Treatment Plan
- Techniques to self-monitor progress
- Positive feedback, encouragement and support from family and health care team
- Patient and family satisfaction with lifestyle changes

The Support Group
- Supplements medical treatment of osteoporosis by educating members to assume greater responsibility for their own health
- Adds a personal dimension to health care by addressing the needs of body, mind, and spirit

Objectives
- Help members realize they are not alone
- Provide information and education
- Support members in their efforts to lead productive lives
- Provide an outlet for feelings
- Provide emotional support and coping strategies

References

1. Bille DA. Developing a philosophy of patient teaching. In: Bille DA (ed), *Practical Approaches to Patient Teaching*. Boston: Little, Brown & Co., 1981;27–33.

2. Gold DT, Drezner MK. Quality of life. In: Riggs BL, Melton LJ III (eds), *Osteoporosis: Etiology, Diagnosis and Management*. Philadelphia: Lippincott-Raven Publishers, 1995;475–486.

3. Horsley JA, Crane J. *Mutual Goal Setting in Patient Care*. New York: Grune & Stratton, Inc., 1992.

4. McClung BL, Overdorf JH. Psychosocial aspects of osteoporosis. In: Rosen CJ (ed), *Osteoporosis: Diagnostic and Therapeutic Principles*. Totowa, NJ: Humana Press Inc., 1996;69–75

5. Pachucki-Hyde L. Innovative patient teaching models from a nursing perspective. Proceeding from the Drug Information Association 2nd Annual Symposium on Osteoporosis Education: Focusing on behavioral change. Philadelphia, PA, April 1997.

34

Resources for Education and Support

Betsy Love McClung

National Osteoporosis Foundation
1150 17th St. NW, Suite 500
Washington, DC 20036
Telephone: General Information (202) 223-2226
Telephone: Support Group Information (312) 464-5110
Fax: (202) 223-2237
E-mail: nofmail@nof.org
Website: http:\\www.nof.org

NIH Osteoporosis and Related Bone Diseases National Resource Center
1150 17th St. NW, Suite 500
Washington, DC 20036
Telephone: (800) 624-2663
E-mail: orbnrc@nof.org
Website: http:\\www.osteo.org

The Osteoporosis Society of Canada
33 Laird Drive
Toronto, Ontario M4G 3S9
Canada
Telephone: (800) 463-6842
Fax: (416) 696-2673
E-mail: osc.osteoporosis.ca
Website: http:\\www.osteoporosis.ca

The Paget Foundation
120 Wall St., Suite 1602
New York, NY 10005
Telephone: (800) 237-2438
Fax: (212) 509-8492
E-mail: pagetfdn.aol.com
Website: http:\\www.paget.org

The Bone and Mineral Manual
Copyright ©1999 by Academic Press
All rights of reproduction in any form reserved.

Osteogenesis Imperfecta Foundation
804 W. Diamond Ave., Suite 210
Gaithersburg, MD 20878
Telephone: (800) 981-2663
Fax: (301) 947-0456
E-mail: bonelink@aol.com
Website: http:\\www.oif.org

The North American Menopause Society
P.O. Box 94527
Cleveland, OH 44101
Telephone: (216) 844-8748; (800) 774-5342
Fax: (216) 844-8708
Website: http:\\www.menopause.org

Appendix A:
National Osteoporosis Foundation Guidelines

Who Should Be Tested for BMD?

- All postmenopausal women under age 65 who have one or more additional risk factors for osteoporosis (besides menopause).
- All women aged 65 and older regardless of additional risk factors.
- Postmenopausal women who present with fractures (to confirm diagnosis and determine disease severity).
- Women who are considering therapy for osteoporosis, if BMD testing would facilitate the decision.
- Women who have been on hormone replacement therapy for prolonged periods.

Who Should Be Treated?

- Women with BMD T-scores below –2 in the absence of osteoporosis risk factors.
- Women with BMD T-scores below –1.5 if other risk factors are present.
- Some patients (i.e., those over 70 with multiple risk factors) are at sufficiently high risk for osteoporosis that treatment is warranted without BMD testing.

From: *Pocket Guide to Prevention and Treatment of Osteoporosis*. National Osteoporosis Foundation, 1998. www.nof.org. Reproduced with permission.

Appendix B:
Bone Mass Measurement Act, 1998

This Benefit Requires Medicare to Cover Bone Mass Measurement for Eligible People in Five Categories:

1. Estrogen-deficient women at clinical risk for osteoporosis
2. Individuals with vertebral abnormalities
3. Long-term recipients of glucocorticoid therapy
4. Individuals with primary hyperparathyroidism
5. Individuals being monitored to assess the response to, or efficacy of an FDA-approved osteoporosis drug.

For additional information, contact the National Osteoporosis Foundation at www.nof.org

Index